W9-CEJ-153

STUDENT STUDY GUIDE TO ACCOMPANY

Maternity Nursing Care

SECOND EDITION

Maternity Nursing Care

SECOND EDITION

Lynna Y. Littleton-Gibbs, RN, PhD, MNN-BC, WHNP-BC, FAANP

Women's Health Nurse Practitioner
Nursing Consultant
Associate Professor of Clinical Nursing (Retired)
School of Nursing
University of Texas Health Science Center at Houston
Houston, Texas

Joan C. Engebretson, RN, DrPH, AHNA-BC

Judy Fred Professor
School of Nursing
University of Texas Health Science Center at Houston
Houston, Texas

Prior edition prepared by
Maxine Lesser, MSN, ARNP

Associate Professor of Nursing
Daytona Beach Community College
Daytona Beach, Florida

and

select materials prepared by
Katherine C. Pearson, BSN, MSN, FNP

and

Ethel Morikis, CMA, BSN, RNC

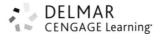

DELMAR
CENGAGE Learning·

Australia • Brazil • Japan • Korea • Mexico • Singapore • Spain • United Kingdom • United States

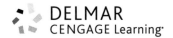

Student Study Guide to Accompany Maternity Nursing Care, Second Edition

Lynna Y. Littleton-Gibbs, Joan C. Engebretson

Vice President, Editorial: Dave Garza

Executive Editor: Stephen Helba

Senior Acquisition Editor: Maureen Rosener

Managing Editor: Marah Bellegarde

Senior Product Manager: Elisabeth F. Williams

Editorial Assistant: Samantha Miller

Vice President, Marketing: Jennifer Baker

Marketing Director: Wendy E. Mapstone

Senior Marketing Manager: Michele McTighe

Marketing Coordinator: Scott A. Chrysler

Production Manager: Andrew Crouth

Content Project Manager: Brooke Greenhouse

Senior Art Director: Jack Pendleton

For product information and technology assistance, contact us at
Cengage Learning Customer & Sales Support, 1-800-354-9706

For permission to use material from this text or product,
submit all requests online at **www.cengage.com/permissions**.
Further permissions questions can be e-mailed to
permissionrequest@cengage.com

Library of Congress Control Number: 2011942529

ISBN-13: 978-1-111-54312-9

ISBN-10: 1-111-54312-7

Delmar
5 Maxwell Drive
Clifton Park, NY 12065-2919
USA

Cengage Learning is a leading provider of customized learning solutions with office locations around the globe, including Singapore, the United Kingdom, Australia, Mexico, Brazil, and Japan. Locate your local office at:
international.cengage.com/region

Cengage Learning products are represented in Canada by Nelson Education, Ltd.

To learn more about Delmar, visit **www.cengage.com/delmar**

Purchase any of our products at your local college store or at our preferred online store **www.cengagebrain.com**

Notice to the Reader

Publisher does not warrant or guarantee any of the products described herein or perform any independent analysis in connection with any of the product information contained herein. Publisher does not assume, and expressly disclaims, any obligation to obtain and include information other than that provided to it by the manufacturer. The reader is expressly warned to consider and adopt all safety precautions that might be indicated by the activities described herein and to avoid all potential hazards. By following the instructions contained herein, the reader willingly assumes all risks in connection with such instructions. The publisher makes no representations or warranties of any kind, including but not limited to, the warranties of fitness for particular purpose or merchantability, nor are any such representations implied with respect to the material set forth herein, and the publisher takes no responsibility with respect to such material. The publisher shall not be liable for any special, consequential, or exemplary damages resulting, in whole or part, from the readers' use of, or reliance upon, this material.

Printed in the United States of America
1 2 3 4 5 6 7 16 15 14 13 12

Contents

Preface

The purpose of the *Student Study Guide to Accompany Maternity Nursing Care*, second edition, is to help you learn, absorb, and retain difficult and often unfamiliar concepts in maternal, neonatal, and women's health nursing. This *Study Guide* helps reinforce the major concepts as you review the central facts of each textbook chapter, and helps you to develop the knowledge and skills you will need to succeed as a nurse in any health care setting. Each chapter of the *Study Guide* covers six areas: Key Terms, Activities, Self- Assessment Quiz, Critical Thinking, Multiple Choice Questions, and Multiple Response Questions.

- Key Terms list the important terminology used in the text. Write down all the definitions you know and then focus on areas where your knowledge base is not as strong.

- Activities are constructed around the key concepts in the textbook chapters. The activities test your understanding and application of those concepts through recognition, recall, and analysis.

- Self-Assessment Quiz includes short answer, matching, and true-false questions that draw on key ideas in the chapter and prepare you to succeed in your examinations.

- Critical Thinking exercises are case-based scenarios which challenge you to synthesize information learned and apply it to new concepts and situations.

- Multiple Choice Questions mimic the format of the NCLEX licensure examination.

- Multiple Response Questions also follow the new NCLEX-style question where multiple answers may be correct.

Suggested responses and rationales are found at the end of the *Study Guide* in the Answer Key.

UNIT 1

Foundations of Maternal, Neonatal, and Women's Health Nursing

CHAPTER 1

Nursing in the Contemporary Health Care System

KEY TERMS

Please define the following terms:

Cost containment

Cultural competence

Cultural competence continuum

Evidence-based practice

Health promotion

Interdisciplinary teams

Managed care

Primary prevention

Risk assessment

Secondary prevention

Tertiary prevention

ACTIVITIES

1. What is the focus of contemporary health care?

2. Immunization is an example of a primary prevention measure. Provide at least two examples of the positive impact of immunization on maternal, neonatal, and women's health.

3. Give an example of risk assessment for a pregnant woman.

4. Describe the nurse's role with home health care agencies.

5. Nurses' roles have expanded and will continue to develop. Describe some roles of the nurse as part of the health care team.

6. Traditionally when dealing with health care issues, the clinician plays the active role and the client remains passive. Explain how these roles are changing.

7. List at least four examples of "Goals for Healthy People 2020."

8. Define how issues related to populations with poor health care, such as access to care, social issues, and the effects of poverty, can be addressed to assist those in need.

9. Appropriate use of technology is often an effective health care measure. Give examples of where technology should be used to diagnose and treat illnesses.

10. Discuss the advantages and disadvantages of managed care.

11. Explain how identification of risk assessment can have a positive impact on maternal and fetal outcomes.

12. Compare multidisciplinary care and interdisciplinary care.

13. Describe some common ethical issues associated with genetic testing.

14. Address the issue of confidentiality and its importance, both legally and ethically, to the client.

15. Describe the importance of responding to health care needs of clients from different cultures.

16. Explain malpractice and how health care providers work to avoid lawsuits.

17. Give examples of types of biological, behavioral, environmental, social, and cultural issues, and alternative and complementary therapies that affect women's health today.

18. Discuss the importance of communication skills between health care providers and clients.

SELF-ASSESSMENT QUIZ

1. True or False

    T   F   Medical advances and technological advances have helped health care costs decrease.

    T   F   Availability of health-related information to the public has expanded.

    T   F   Emphasis toward health interventions has shifted from large hospitals to the community.

    T   F   Health maintenance organizations offer the consumer more options.

    T   F   Risk assessment is used to identify women who have factors that contribute to having negative fetal outcomes.

    T   F   A good relationship with a client is not a major source of malpractice claims.

    T   F   Certification is required for a nurse to become credentialed.

    T   F   In the current health care system, it is not sufficient for the practicing nurse to simply follow the physician's orders.

2. Identify new types of care delivery that are emerging to move clients from the hospital to the home or other community settings.

3. List the three types of managed care programs that provide insurance coverage for clients.

4. Describe telemedicine and its importance in health care.

5. Describe critical thinking skills.

6. When is the use of RhoGam indicated?

7. Name the important considerations to include in nursing documentation.

8. Suggest two transitional times for women that are significantly affected by cultural beliefs.

9. Name some specialties within maternal nursing that require certification.

CRITICAL THINKING

1. Discuss the Patient Protection and Affordable Care Act (PPAC) and its effects on mothers and infants.

2. How might limited resources affect women's health?

MULTIPLE CHOICE

1. Which of the following statements is true about ultrasonography?

   A. Health care providers started using ultrasounds in the 1940s to detect problems with fetal development.
   B. An ultrasound is often used to detect the presence of a brain hemorrhage in newborn infants.
   C. Ultrasonography is only conducted by certified and trained ultrasound technologists.
   D. An ultrasound can be a valid substitute for some other types of tests, such as amniocentesis.

2. Medical errors have gained attention as being major causes of morbidity and mortality. Which of the following is a true statement about medical errors?

   A. Medical errors are typically caused by incompetence on the part of the health care provider.
   B. Reducing the occurrences of medical errors should be the exclusive effort of hospital administration.
   C. Errors of execution occur when the intended action is incorrect.
   D. The single most important way a patient can help to prevent medical errors is to be an active member of the health care team.

3. Nurses can reduce the risk of becoming a defendant in a lawsuit by:

   A. developing caring relationships with clients
   B. contacting their hospital administration for insurance coverage in case of a complaint
   C. following all guidelines and practices for patient care in the same method as was taught in nursing school
   D. taking on more assignments because it is no longer safe to delegate to unlicensed personnel

4. The minimally accepted standards for the practice of professional nursing within each state is known as:

   A. certification
   B. credentialing

   C. specialization
   D. licensure

5. Those beliefs and values that guide behavior and are integrated into daily life are called:

   A. cultural competencies
   B. self-reflections

   C. cultural heritage
   D. personal awareness

MULTIPLE RESPONSE

1. The nurse involved in maternal, neonatal, and women's health care must be aware of the many trends that affect today's health care system, including which of the following? Select all that apply.

   A. an increase in births outside of hospitals
   B. more women choosing physicians over midwives for care
   C. cost reduction due to decreased hospital stays
   D. community maternity facilities in major cities seeing more high-risk clients
   E. an increase in labor inductions and a decrease in Lamaze classes

2. The Agenda for Research on Women's Health for the 21st Century has explored some differences between women's and men's health. Which of the following social issues are true regarding disparities between women's and men's health? Select all that apply.

   A. Women use health care services less often than men.
   B. Men often live longer than women.
   C. Women are more eager to support the health of their families than men.
   D. Greater numbers of men live at low-income or poverty levels than women.
   E. Women are often more receptive to health education than men.

3. Providing risk assessment is essential for which of the following reasons? Select all that apply.

   A. Risk assessments may screen for eating disorders, domestic violence, or cancer.
   B. Risk assessments provide care for infants who are unable to discuss signs or symptoms of illness.
   C. Risk assessments promote cost-effective measures that adhere to the institution's budget.
   D. Risk assessments provide care to reduce complications during procedures.
   E. Risk assessments are valuable because they are often repeated with each visit.

CHAPTER 2

Theoretical Perspectives on the Childbearing Family

KEY TERMS

Please define the following terms:

Blended family

Cohabitation

Communal family

Crisis

Cultural competence continuum

Developmental crisis

Dyads

Extended family

Family structure

Nuclear family

Reconstituted family

Situational crisis

Transitions

ACTIVITIES

1. Identify and describe various forms of family structures.
   Traditional or nuclear family

   Childless dyad

   Extended family

   Communal family

   Unmarried heterosexual family or cohabitation

   Homosexual family

   Single-parent family

   Reconstituted or blended family

2. Discuss psychosocial resources available for single-parent families.

3. List the basic functions of the family. Discuss some potential implications to society when the family is unable to meet the basic needs of its members.

4. Describe the influence of noncustodial parents.

5. List at least three potential problems that may arise in a blended family.

6. List several nursing implications for the childbearing family.

7. Explain how the change in the role of women has affected family structure.

8. Why should the nurse assess family dynamics before designing a plan of care for the family as clients?

SELF-ASSESSMENT QUIZ

1. True or False

    T   F   Traditional family models may be used to identify the reconstituted family.

    T   F   Stepfamilies typically have fewer stressors than traditional families.

    T   F   Extended families provide additional support systems.

    T   F   There are no support resources available for single-parent families.

    T   F   Sexuality may be a source of stress in any type of family.

2. List and discuss some tips that might be useful for working with blended families.

3. Discuss the possible impact of continuous support during the birth process to the laboring mother.

4. Discuss appropriate nursing interventions during the birth experience that can assist the father with his participation in the birth process.

CRITICAL THINKING

1. Sara and David were happily anticipating the birth of their first child. Unfortunately, Sara went into labor at 22 weeks' gestation and delivered a tiny stillborn baby girl. Both parents were devastated by this event but appeared to have completely different reactions. Sara wanted to hold her baby daughter. You observed Sara tenderly gazing into her daughter's face and softly talking about all the good times they would have had together. David reacted quite differently. He appeared angry and upset with the health care team. His concerns focused on how and why this happened, and he demanded to know what went wrong.

   It is critical for the nurse caring for this family to provide culturally sensitive care while assisting this family through the stages of grieving.

   a. List the stages of grieving by Kübler-Ross.

   b. Which stages are Sara and David experiencing at this time?

   c. List appropriate nursing interventions when providing care for the family experiencing perinatal loss.

2. Ms. Jiminez is a single mother with two children ages seven months and three years. She has missed the last two scheduled well-baby visits for her seven-month-old. The nurse practitioner responsible for the baby's care is concerned and phones Ms. Jiminez at home. Ms. Jiminez explains that she no longer has a car and would need to take two buses to come to the clinic. Not only would this be very difficult with a baby, but it would cause her to miss an entire day of work.

   Poor access is an important factor in health care. Discuss some possible measures or suggestions that you could implement to assist this client and her family.

3. In your opinion, what kind of influence does prime-time television have on the American family, if any?

MULTIPLE CHOICE

1. The "S" in the NURSE acronym used to describe a nursing approach to enable women to address the emotional challenges of the postpartum period stands for:

   A. symptoms   C. standardization
   B. spirituality   D. social functions

2. Which of the following is true about the experience of a father surrounding the birth encounter?

   A. The father typically perceives the reality of the child during the pregnancy period.
   B. The father's experience in the birth should closely resemble the mother's through his participation.
   C. The father's experiences are influenced by attitudes of the health care providers who interact with him during the birth experience.
   D. The father's needs are typically addressed on an individual basis, separate from the needs of the mother.

3. The concept on the cultural competence continuum that ignores the cultural strengths of the family, encourages assimilation, and blames the family for not "fitting in" is known as:

   A. cultural proficiency
   B. cultural pre-competence
   C. cultural destructiveness
   D. cultural blindness

4. A type of family that forms because the earlier marriage or partnership of one or both of the parents ended is called a(n):

   A. reconstituted family
   B. cohabitating family
   C. extended family
   D. communal family

5. Which of the following data would you not expect to be gathered during assessment of the childbearing family?

   A. the patient's values and beliefs about parenting
   B. previous experiences with infant and child care
   C. the interactions between the grandparents and the father of the baby
   D. social resources, such as housing needs, income and extended family support

MULTIPLE RESPONSE

1. Family systems theories describe the relationship of the individual and the multiple forces with which the individual interacts throughout life. Which of the following are concepts that describe family systems? Select all that apply.

   A. A change in one member of the family impacts parents more than children within the family.
   B. The nuclear family and its traditional structure equates with idealized function.
   C. The family as a whole is greater than, and different from, the sum of its parts.
   D. Families create a balance between change and stability.
   E. Family members' behaviors are better understood from the perspective of circular, rather than linear, causality.

2. Which of the following are associated with maternal role development and transition to parenting? Select all that apply.

    A. social support
    B. age
    C. breastfeeding
    D. self-esteem
    E. marital status

3. For the birthing woman, a deviation from expectations about the birthing process can create which of the following? Select all that apply.

    A. denial
    B. a sense of unfulfillment
    C. loss of integrity related to body boundaries
    D. feelings of rejection
    E. irritation

CHAPTER 3

Complementary and Alternative Therapies

KEY TERMS

Please define the following terms:

Acupressure

Acupuncture

Allopathy

Alternative therapies

Ayurvedic medicine

Biomedicine

Chi

Chi gong

Complementary therapies (CTs)

Culture

Dosha

Healing systems

Holism

Integrated medicine

Meridian

Moxibustion

Phytotherapy

Prana

Vitalism

ACTIVITIES

1. List the seven classifications of complementary and alternative practices.

2. Discuss and compare the differences and similarities among the five traditional healing systems.

   Traditional Chinese medicine

   Ayurvedic medicine

   Yoga

Shamanic healing

Ritual healing

3. Identify and describe the differences in the four approaches of self-healing.
   Osteopathic medicine

   Chiropractic medicine

   Homeopathy

   Naturopathy

4. Name six herbs to be avoided during pregnancy.

5. Name 12 herbs to be avoided if lactating.

6. List nine herbs that should not be taken without medical supervision.

7. Identify the herbs that are contraindicated in clients who have the following:
   Allergy to daisies

   Prescription for anticoagulant therapy

   Diabetes

   Hypertension

   Allergy to ragweed

SELF-ASSESSMENT QUIZ

1. Match the healing system with its definition.

_____ Traditional Chinese medicine

    A. Healing practice that may involve physical manipulation, ingestion or application of natural substances, and supernormal actions

_____ Yoga

    B. Needs to be approached in the context of the religious belief and practice

_____ Shamanic healing

    C. Is holistic and based on the concept of balance and a vital life force

_____ Ritual healing

    D. Based on interrelatedness between the whole person and nature

_____ Ayurvedic medicine

    E. A philosophy of ethics and personal discipline

2. True or False

  T   F   The incidence of medical schools adding a CAM course is increasing.

  T   F   Neglecting to ask the client about the use of herbs, vitamins, or other dietary supplements could lead to harmful drug interactions.

  T   F   Ginkgo biloba, grape seed extract, and bilberry possess antiplatelet activity.

  T   F   Ginger, garlic, and ginseng may interfere with anticoagulant or antiplatelet medications.

  T   F   Registered nurses with a baccalaureate degree can become certified as holistic nurses.

3. If a client has an adverse effect or drug reaction to an herbal product, should it be reported? If so, where?

4. Doctors of osteopathy have what additional training?

5. What herb may increase the size of cataracts?

CRITICAL THINKING

1. Your neighbor is undergoing chemotherapy for colon cancer. She is discouraged by her lack of progress with the traditional care she is receiving. While surfing the Internet she found a supposedly natural product that promises to cure her cancer. She is desperate and wants your advice. How would you respond?

2. Research the use of moxibustion in obstetrics.

3. In many cases, clients do not tell their providers that they are using complementary therapies. What do you believe the reason(s) for this might be?

MULTIPLE CHOICE

1. The essence of who we are as human beings and the process of discovering purpose, meaning, and inner strength throughout life's journey is known as:

   A. religion
   B. vitalism
   C. spirituality
   D. holism

2. Which of the following is a type of mind-body therapy?

   A. cognitive repatterning
   B. healing touch
   C. transcutaneous electrical nerve stimulation (TENS)
   D. magnetic healing

3. A type of herb used during perimenopause that reduces luteinizing hormone production and may have mild estrogenic activity is called:

   A. chaste berry
   B. black cohosh
   C. motherwort
   D. sage

4. The practice that focuses on a particular philosophy of life, rather than a specific disease treatment, is known as:

   A. osteopathy
   B. allopathy
   C. naturopathy
   D. homeopathy

5. A body work technique that uses self-induced movements to recognize and unlearn some types of harmful physical and mental habits is called:

   A. rolfing
   B. myofascial release
   C. craniosacral manipulation
   D. Trager

MULTIPLE RESPONSE

1. Body work techniques are types of physical manipulation that require a trained therapist. Which of the following are types of body work techniques? Select all that apply.

   A. massage therapy
   B. Pilates
   C. rolfing
   D. craniosacral manipulations
   E. calisthenics

2. Energy-based therapies focus on the energy field rather than the physical body. Which of the following are considered to be energy-based therapies? Select all that apply.

   A. Reiki
   B. therapeutic touch
   C. healing touch
   D. phytotherapy
   E. autogenic training

3. What are some precautions to consider when using herbal therapy? Select all that apply.

   A. Ephedra is a major component of many weight loss products on the market today and clients should carefully consider its side effects.
   B. The levels of active ingredients within herbal preparations can vary with growing conditions.
   C. Although standardized manufacturing exists, the FDA has not proposed any regulatory standards.
   D. Some plant ingredients are toxic.
   E. Not all parts of the plant have medicinal action or similar effects.

CHAPTER 4

Ethics, Laws, and Standards of Care

KEY TERMS

Please define the following terms:

Autonomy

Beneficence

Categorical imperative

Civil law

Code

Criminal law

Deontology

Dilemma

Doctrine of the Golden Mean

Due care

Ethic of care

Ethical dilemmas

Ethics

Fidelity

Harm

Informed consent

Justice

Law

Liability

Malpractice

Material principles of justice

Moral distress

Negligence

Nonmaleficence

Paternalism

Prima facie

Standards of care

Tort

Universalizability

Utilitarianism

Veracity

Virtue

Virtue ethics

ACTIVITIES

1. Compare and contrast laws and ethics.

2. List all the people you believe should be part of an ethics committee in a hospital setting.

3. Contrast basic ethical perspectives.

	Definition	Positive Aspects	Negative Aspects	Examples
Utilitarianism				
Deontology				
Virtue ethics				

Nursing ethics

Holistic ethics

---

4. Give one example that could be encountered in your clinical setting for each of the following major ethical principles:

Autonomy

Nonmaleficence

Beneficence

Justice

Veracity

Fidelity

5. Propose a brief client education plan for informing a person about advance directives. Be sure important areas are covered.

6. With your lab partner, apply the ethical decision-making framework to examine one of the following maternal-child dilemmas:

Abortion

Maternal-fetal conflict

Genetic mapping

Selective abortion

Surrogate motherhood

Female circumcision

7. List four questions nurses may ask themselves to determine the scope of practice.

8. How would you approach a client at high risk for obstetric complications to ask whether she has completed an advance directive? Practice discussing this issue with your lab partner.

SELF-ASSESSMENT QUIZ

1. What standards of care are utilized for women's health?

2. True or False
T	F	The Board of Nursing for each state establishes regulations governing nursing practice.
T	F	Criminal law is regulated by the Board of Nursing for each state.
T	F	A tort is a civil wrong.
T	F	Malpractice occurs when there is negligence caused by the failure to act as a competent professional would under similar circumstances.
T	F	A standard of care is a document developed by professional groups to establish a level of practice agreed on by members of the profession.

CRITICAL THINKING

1. At 14 weeks' gestation, the client is informed that her unborn baby has Down syndrome. She and her husband are brokenhearted. Her husband wants her to have an elective abortion, but the client feels very conflicted. They come to you, the nurse, for advice. How would you respond?

2. When you report for work in the nursing unit, you discover that two nurses called in sick, and the staffing level is below the standard for the unit. The nurse manager tells you that times are tough, and with the nursing shortage, this kind of problem will occur more often. She informs you that you have a duty to the clients and the hospital to do the best you can. What are your responsibilities and how can you respond to this situation?

MULTIPLE CHOICE

1. _____ is the concept of preventing intentional or unintentional harm to others.

   A. Beneficence
   B. Nonmaleficence
   C. Due care
   D. Justice

2. A pregnant client in labor wants to deliver her baby without the use of medication. The nurse responds by saying, "Believe me, when the time comes, you will want an epidural. Let me get you the consent." The nurse is demonstrating the principle of _____.

   A. beneficence
   B. fidelity
   C. autonomy
   D. paternalism

3. The "B" in SBAR, an approach that facilitates communication of pertinent information, stands for _____.

   A. background
   B. benefits
   C. backup
   D. build

4. Which of the following is NOT a suggested question that nurses may ask to determine the acceptability of their practices?

   A. Is the activity consistent with the state's Nurse Practice Act and rules and regulations of the Board of Nursing?
   B. Does the practice adhere to the nurse's personal belief system?
   C. Is the activity supported by research or in the scope and standards of practice statements?
   D. Would a reasonable and prudent nurse perform the activity in this setting?

5. The categorical imperative, or supreme rule that should govern actions, was first proposed by:

   A. W. D. Ross
   B. Aristotle
   C. Immanuel Kant
   D. Gadow

MULTIPLE RESPONSE

1. Which of the following would be a common step used in a framework designed to reflect on difficult ethical situations? Select all that apply.

   A. gathering information about the situation
   B. notifying social services about patient non-compliance
   C. applying principles and values to guide reasoning
   D. writing down directions for the patient to follow
   E. informing the physician of the need to be involved

2. Which of the following are competing values that may be present in maternal-fetal conflicts? Select all that apply.

   A. autonomy of the pregnant woman
   B. protection of the common good
   C. sovereignty of the physician
   D. protection of the nurse
   E. protection of the fetus

3. During pregnancy, women infected with untreated human immunodeficiency virus (HIV) may transmit the infection to their unborn child. Why is prenatal testing an important issue in this matter? Select all that apply.

   A. The client can understand how long she will be hospitalized.
   B. The nurse will be aware of the need for universal precautions.
   C. The client can start antiretroviral therapy, which could reduce transmission to the fetus.
   D. Knowledge of the virus may help to reduce perinatal complications.
   E. The client and nurse will be aware that pregnancy may increase personal risk by altering cell-mediated immunity.

UNIT 2
Health Care of Women Across the Lifespan

CHAPTER 5

Promoting Women's Health

KEY TERMS

Please define the following terms:

Acquaintance rape

Adolescence

Anorexia nervosa

Anovulatory cycle

Basal metabolism

Binge eating

Body mass index (BMI)

Bulimia nervosa

Calorie

Corpus luteum

Daily reference values (DRVs)

Date rape

Dietary Guidelines for Americans

Gonadotropin-releasing hormone (Gn-RH)

Heme iron

Hypochromic anemia

Hypothalamic-pituitary-ovarian axis

Insoluble fiber

Intimate partner violence (IPV)

Menarche

Menopause

Microcytic anemia

MyPlate

Non-heme iron

Nutrient dense

Nutrition Facts Food Label

Obesity

Osteopenia

Osteoporosis

Ovulation

Perimenopause

Perpetrator

Puberty

Rape

Recommended dietary allowances (RDAs)

Reference daily intakes (RDIs)

Soluble fiber

Stranger rape

Stress incontinence

Tanner stages

Thelarche

Wife rape

ACTIVITIES

1. Define the three phases of the menstrual cycle.

2. Discuss two examples of primary prevention measures for adolescent females.

3. Differentiate between perimenopause and menopause.

4. Discuss at least three specific physiologic changes that occur during menopause.

5. What factors contribute to osteoporosis?

6. Propose a client education plan for a woman to prevent or treat osteoporosis.

7. Discuss the appropriate anticipatory guidance for a client who is approaching menopause. Include the expected physiologic changes that may occur in her body.

8. How has the midlife woman's perception of life changed in the past 20 years?

9. Compare psychosocial changes, cultural influences, and self-care for women throughout the life span.

	Psychosocial Changes	Cultural Influences	Self-Care Considerations
Adolescence			
Young Adulthood			
Perimenopause			
Mature Years			

10. Discuss ChooseMyPlate.

11. Find two food labels and identify the following:

	Label 1	**Label 2**
Serving size	_____	_____
Recommended dietary allowance	_____	_____
Total fat	_____	_____
Cholesterol	_____	_____
Sodium	_____	_____
Total carbohydrates	_____	_____
Dietary fiber	_____	_____
Sugars	_____	_____
Protein	_____	_____
Vitamin A	_____	_____
Vitamin C	_____	_____
Calcium	_____	_____
Iron	_____	_____

12. Complete the table for DRVs.

Substance	% Of Total Calories
Total Carbohydrate	
Protein	
Total Fat	
Saturated Fat	

13. Compare the dietary needs of women in the following age groups:

Age Group	Specific Dietary Recommendations
Adolescent	
Adult	
Childbearing	
Elderly	

14. List the common complications of anorexia nervosa.

15. List the anatomic and physiologic changes associated with bulimia nervosa.

16. Describe the diagnostic criteria for binge eating.

17. Explain the benefits of exercise for women throughout the life span.

18. What anticipatory guidance questions can the nurse ask a woman who has survived sexual assault? What are the phases of rape trauma syndrome?

19. List the steps to assess a woman's immediate danger and formulate a safety plan.

20. What responsibility does the nurse have when caring for a client who has been a victim of abuse? Are there any differences in responsibilities depending on the age of the client?

21. Find two resources on the Web related to domestic violence.

22. Research the role of a sexual assault nurse examiner.

SELF-ASSESSMENT QUIZ

1. What is the mean age of menarche?

2. Which is the leading cause of death for women?
   Breast cancer

   Heart disease

   Ovarian cancer

   Stress

3. What is the most common cause of dysfunctional uterine bleeding?

4. True or False

 T   F   Phytochemical antioxidants include vitamins A, D, E, and K.

 T   F   Following dietary recommendations can help prevent osteoporosis.

 T   F   Good nutrition does not affect any types of cancer.

 T   F   Depression is related to physiology as well as the social and economic factors that women face in their mature years.

5. What are the two most prevalent risk factors for being an abuser?

CRITICAL THINKING

1. In your role as the school nurse, you are conducting routine health screening exams. One of your students is Maria. Maria is a thin, well-groomed, attractive 15-year-old girl. She is bright and vivacious, but after examining her, you realize that she is very underweight. When you call her mother to discuss your concerns, her mother tells you that she is worried about her daughter as well. She tells you that ever since Maria was chosen for the cheerleading team, she has been obsessed with dieting and exercising.

   a. What medical diagnosis do you suspect?

   b. What further questions would you ask Maria at this time?

   c. You are reasonably sure that Maria is suffering from anorexia nervosa. What suggestions or recommendations would you have for Maria and her mother at this time?

2. While assisting the client in getting ready for a pelvic examination, you observe bruising on the client's abdomen and breast. The client appears uncomfortable with your observation and tells you that she took a bad fall and is always clumsy. You suspect abuse.

   a. What additional questions would you ask at this time?

   b. If the client insists her bruises are the result of falls, what, if anything, could you do?

   c. List at least three specific goals designed to keep a woman safe from physical abuse.

MULTIPLE CHOICE

1. Which nutrient promotes blood formation and aids in the synthesis of RNA and DNA?

   A. vitamin D
   B. vitamin B_{12}
   C. folate
   D. calcium

2. Prior to ovulation, an increase in estrogen causes a surge of luteinizing hormone to be released from which part of the body?

   A. the ovary
   B. the hypothalamus
   C. the pituitary gland
   D. the uterus

3. An involuntary discharge of urine with a cough, sneeze, or laughter owing to the loss of muscular support at the neck of the urethra is known as _____.

   A. urge incontinence
   B. overflow incontinence
   C. functional incontinence
   D. stress incontinence

4. A publication that provides guidance on diet and health to the general population with practical recommendations is called _____.

   A. Dietary Guidelines for Americans
   B. MyPlate
   C. Nutrition Facts Food Label
   D. reference daily intakes

5. An essential nutrient responsible for transporting other nutrients in the body and regulating body temperature is known as _____.

   A. potassium
   B. fiber
   C. water
   D. sodium

MULTIPLE RESPONSE

1. Thiedke and Rosenfeld outlined some of the sociologic tasks of older women, including which of the following? Select all that apply.

   A. adjusting to retirement and its reduced income
   B. establishing satisfactory physical living arrangements
   C. adjusting to increased bone and joint pain
   D. adopting and adapting to social roles in a flexible way
   E. adjusting to mood changes, including depression

2. Family violence patterns often follow typical phases. Which of the following are phases of family violence? Select all that apply.

   A. forgiveness phase
   B. tension-building phase
   C. acute battering phase
   D. regression phase
   E. honeymoon phase

3. Vitamin D is important for the absorption of calcium and phosphorus for good bone mineralization. Which of the following foods are good sources of vitamin D? Select all that apply.

   A. fish liver oils
   B. meat
   C. legumes
   D. yeast
   E. raisins

CHAPTER 6

Health Care Issues and Reproductive Concerns

KEY TERMS

Please define the following terms:

Amenorrhea

Birth rate

Cancer

Carcinoma in situ

Cervical infection

Dysfunctional uterine bleeding (DUB)

Dysmenorrhea

Endometriosis

False discharge

Fertility rate

Fibrocystic changes

Fibroid tumors

Health promotion

Health protection

Invasive breast cancer

Invasive cancer

Lactation discharge

Life expectancy

Localized breast cancer

Mastectomy

Menopause

Metastatic breast cancer

Morbidity rate

Mortality rate

Nipple discharge

Osteoporosis

Pap smear

Pathologic discharge

Pelvic inflammatory disease (PID)

Pelvic relaxation

Physiologic discharge

Polycystic ovary syndrome

Premenstrual syndrome (PMS)

Primary amenorrhea

Primary dysmenorrhea

Screening

Secondary amenorrhea

Secondary dysmenorrhea

Vaginal infection

ACTIVITIES

1. How has women's health been affected by history?

2. Discuss how the role of the midwife has evolved in reproductive care.

3. Explain factors that influence women's health throughout the life span.

4. Describe the relationship between women's health and research.

5. Discuss the relationship between education and health status.

6. Why are women with heart disease less likely than men to seek medical attention? How does this affect morbidity and mortality rates?

7. Complete the following table for primary prevention health measures.

Disease	Incidence	Risk Factors	S/SX	Primary Prevention	Secondary Prevention
CV disease					
Lung cancer					
Breast cancer					
Colon and rectal cancer					
Cervical cancer					
Endometrial cancer					

Ovarian cancer

Osteoporosis

_____

8. Propose an educational plan to help a client quit smoking. Include the benefits of not smoking.

9. Create a client education plan to teach breast self-examination. Practice teaching to a lab partner.

10. How are women affected by substance abuse?

11. Discuss preventive services for the following activities:

    Counseling

    Immunizations

    Screening

12. Compare and contrast primary and secondary amenorrhea.

SELF-ASSESSMENT QUIZ

1. Which race and gender has the longest life expectancy?

2. List four missions of the Office of Research on Women's Health established in 1990 by the National Institutes of Health.

3. What is the leading cause of death for both men and women?

4. List five risk factors for osteoporosis.

5. List five risk factors for breast cancer.

6. What are the most common risk factors for PID?

CRITICAL THINKING

1. Mrs. Dreblinki is a 41-year-old woman who has come to see her doctor for a routine physical exam. Review her assessment data.

Subjective Data

Client reports smoking a pack a day for the last 10 years.

Client reports a family history of heart disease.

Client enjoys cooking high-fat, traditional Spanish foods.

Client enjoys exercise and walks several miles each day.

Client reports having a high-stress job.

Objective Data

Her physical exam reveals that she is 20% above her ideal weight (BMI 26.1).

Blood pressure 120/80.

Blood glucose 77 mg/dl.

All other labs are within normal limits.

Lung sounds clear throughout.

a. What are Mrs. Dreblinki's risk factors for cardiac disease?

b. What lifestyle behaviors would you encourage Mrs. Dreblinki to continue?

c. What lifestyle changes or modifications would you encourage Mrs. Dreblinki to make?

d. What nursing diagnosis would you list as your highest priority?

e. Write at least three nursing interventions to assist Mrs. Dreblinki in reducing her cardiac risk factors.

2. List and discuss therapeutic interventions for PMS.

MULTIPLE CHOICE

1. A diagnosis of stage two breast cancer through the TNM staging method, would be considered what type of breast cancer?

   A. metastatic breast cancer
   B. malignant breast cancer
   C. invasive breast cancer
   D. localized breast cancer

2. A practice that includes consideration of adequate nutrition intake, development and maintenance of physical fitness, stress management skills, optimal bone density, and avoidance of hazardous substances is known as health _____.

   A. protection
   B. promotion
   C. prevention
   D. status

3. In 2007, heart disease accounted for over _____ deaths among women and was the first leading cause of death for this group.

   A. 30,000
   B. 300,000
   C. 3 million
   D. 30 million

4. A _____ mastectomy removes the breast, lymph nodes from the axilla, and pectoral muscles.

   A. modified radical mastectomy
   B. simple mastectomy
   C. subcutaneous mastectomy
   D. radical mastectomy

5. Which of the following is not a risk factor for osteoporosis?

   A. obesity
   B. smoking
   C. excess salt intake
   D. premature menopause

MULTIPLE RESPONSE

1. Which of the following are sociocultural factors that threaten the physical and mental well being of women? Select all that apply.

   A. promoting reproductive choices
   B. living longer than men
   C. limited access to health care services
   D. more difficulty obtaining health insurance
   E. experiencing higher rates of illness

2. Which of the following factors have been major factors in increasing the life expectancy of women? Select all that apply.

   A. public sanitation
   B. analgesic therapy
   C. immunizations
   D. advances in maternity care
   E. biomedicine

3. Which of the following are considered to be risk factors for colorectal cancer? Select all that apply.

   A. ulcerative colitis
   B. personal history of lung cancer
   C. smoking
   D. age over 50
   E. low-fiber diet

UNIT 3
Human Reproduction

CHAPTER 7

Reproduction, Sexuality, Infertility, and Family Planning

KEY TERMS

Please define the following terms:

Abortion

Anovulatory

Cervical cap

Coitus interruptus

Contraception

Corpus luteum

Desire phase

Diaphragm

Emergency contraception

Endometriosis

Endometrium

Estrogen

Excitement phase

Family planning

Follicle-stimulating hormone (FSH)

Follicular phase

Galactorrhea

Germ cells

Gonadal

Gonadotropin-releasing hormone (Gn-RH)

Graafian follicle

Human chorionic gonadotropin (hCG)

Hydrocele

Hypothalamic-pituitary-gonadal axis

Implantable contraception

Infertility

Injectable contraceptive

Leydig cells

Libido

Luteal phase

Luteinizing hormone (LH)

Menarche

Menopause

Menses

Menstrual phase

Mittelschmerz

Neurohormonal

Orgasmic phase

Ovulation

Ovulation prediction

Perimenopause

Plateau phase

Precocious

Progesterone

Proliferative phase

Prostaglandins

Refractory period

Resolution phase

Secretory phase

Seminiferous tubules

Serial monogamy

Sexual dysfunction

Sperm capacitation

Spermatogenesis

Spermatozoa

Spermicide

Spinnbarkeit

Sterilization

Testosterone

Tubal ligation

Vaginal ring

Varicocele

Vasectomy

ACTIVITIES

1. State the factors that may cause early or delayed menarche.

2. Describe the menstrual cycle (timing).

3. Define the following endometrial activity:
   Menstrual phase

   Proliferative phase

   Secretary phase

4. Explain spinnbarkeit.

5. Describe ovulation.

6. Explain hormone regulation in the female and the problems that could result.

7. Describe the different phases of the human sexual response:
   Desire phase

   Excitement phase

   Plateau phase

   Orgasmic phase

   Resolution phase

   Refractory period

8. Identify and describe the two physiologic sexual changes women experience as they age.

9. Define infertility and the associated financial and psychological costs.

10. Describe the factors affecting female fertility.

11. Describe the factors affecting male fertility.

12. Outline an assessment of the infertile couple.

13. Differentiate between advantages and disadvantages of the tools used to assess infertility.

14. Express your thoughts and feelings about the ethics of freezing or destroying embryos.

15. Indicate the order in which females rank risk factors in reproductive decisions.

16. Discuss the importance of the nurse in understanding the cultural and social beliefs of women in decision making regarding reproduction.

17. Summarize the spiritual and religious influences in reproductive decision making.

18. Differentiate between the ability to have freedom and the inability to make choices in reproduction.

19. Describe the three decisive points that are relative to contraceptive use:

    Sexual activity

    Preventive contraception

    Emergency contraception

20. Discuss the knowledge necessary to make informed reproductive decisions.

21. Describe the nurse's role in assisting a woman in making choices in contraception.

22. Describe the pharmacology and dosage of the following types of combined oral contraceptives.

Type	Pharmacology	Dosage
Monophasic		
Biphasic		
Multiphasic		

23. Discuss the 11 non-contraceptive benefits of oral contraceptives.

24. Use the following categories to describe combined oral contraceptives:
    Pharmacology

    Efficacy

    Benefits and risks

    Indications

    Contraindications

    Side effects

25. List the absolute contraindications to the use of combined oral contraceptives.

26. List the drug interactions that clients must be informed of with combined oral contraceptives.

27. Use the following categories to discuss intrauterine methods of contraception:

Composition

Mechanism of action

Efficacy

Benefits and risks

Indications

Contraindications

Side effects

28. Use the following categories to discuss the vaginal ring:

Types of

Composition

Mechanism of action

Benefits and risks

Indications

Contraindications

Side effects

29. Compare the following barrier methods of contraception:

	Condom	Diaphragm	Cervical Cap	Spermicide
Mechanism of action				
Benefits and risks				
Indications				
Contraindications				
Side effects				

30. Use the following categories to discuss implantable methods of contraception:

    Composition

    Mechanism of action

    Efficacy

    Benefits and risks

    Indications

    Contraindications

    Side effects

31. Use the following categories to discuss injectable methods of contraception:

    Mechanism of action

Benefits and risks

Indications

Contraindications

Side effects

32. Compare the two natural family planning methods:

	Coitus Interruptus	Ovulation Prediction
Mechanism of action		
Benefits and risks		
Indications		
Contraindications		

33. Compare the different types of emergency contraception:

	Combined Oral Contraceptive	Progestin-Only Pills	Intrauterine Devices
Mechanism of action			
Efficacy			
Benefits and risks			
Indications			
Contraindications			
Side effects			

34. Compare the sterilization methods for females and males:

	Females	Males
Benefits and risks		
Indications		
Contraindications		
Side effects		
Effectiveness		

SELF-ASSESSMENT QUIZ

1. What is the term used to describe the onset of menstrual bleeding?

2. Describe the onset and determining factors for completion of menopause.

3. Explain sexual dysfunction.

4. Explain the acronym PLISSIT.

5. Define infertility.

6. Define endometriosis and how it is associated with infertility.

7. Women often make choices in their reproductive decisions on what basis?

8. Name the two types of contraceptive methods.

9. Name the three basic types of oral contraceptives.

10. When a woman uses combined oral contraceptives, she may acquire a reduced risk for a major disease for a long period. Explain this.

11. Progestin-only contraceptives are indicated for which type of clients?

12. State the major problem with the use of the minipill.

13. State the most important fact in the use of the intrauterine method of contraception.

14. List four misconceptions in the use of intrauterine devices.

15. Under what indications must a client be re-measured for a diaphragm?

16. List items of importance a client must be informed of when utilizing a diaphragm.

17. List the nursing instruction to the client using a cervical cap.

18. Summarize the benefits and risks of implantable contraception.

19. Name and describe the two types of family planning methods.

20. When is the appropriate time in the menstrual cycle for a female to have a sterilization?

21. Name the types of sterilization for women and men.

22. True or False

   T   F   Women rank protection from sexually transmitted diseases as the most important health factor in pregnancy protection.

   T   F   The use of contraception is lower in couples that have just met than in couples with an established relationship.

   T   F   Each opportunity for intercourse is a decision point. Women have a choice regarding it.

   T   F   The effect of sterilization on males and females is immediate.

   T   F   Development of sperm in the testes takes approximately 70 days.

   T   F   Ejaculated sperm can live for four to five days in the female genital tract.

   T   F   Serial monogamy is the practice of having numerous sexual partners at a time.

   T   F   Women maintain sexual desires even after menopause.

CRITICAL THINKING

1. Discuss the dramatic changes in American culture involving the meaning of sexuality, and discuss the impact of modern contraception on sexuality.

MULTIPLE CHOICE

1. The phase of endometrial activity which describes the endometrium from the end of menses through ovulation is called the _____.

   A. menstrual phase   C. proliferative phase
   B. secretory phase   D. implantation phase

2. A type of tool used to assess infertility that determines if the uterine cavity and fallopian tubes are open and healthy is known as a(n) _____.

    A. laparoscopy
    B. hysterosalpingogram
    C. endometrial biopsy
    D. ultrasound

3. Which of the following is a potential benefit of using a cervical cap?

    A. It can be left in place for up to 4 hours after intercourse.
    B. It secretes hormones that increase viscosity of the cervical mucous.
    C. Unlike a diaphragm, it does not need to be fitted by a health care provider.
    D. Additional spermicide does not need to be applied with each act of intercourse.

4. Which of the following statements explains spinnbarkeit?

    A. the enlargement of the selected follicle during ovulation
    B. pain in the lower abdomen during the time of ovulation
    C. increased elasticity of cervical mucous during ovulation
    D. the remnant of the dominant follicle left behind after ovulation

5. The "P" of the PLISSIT model that has been identified as useful for discussing sexual concerns stands for _____.

    A. permission
    B. pregnancy
    C. positive
    D. primary

MULTIPLE RESPONSE

1. Which of the following medications are used for the treatment of ovarian disorders? Select all that apply.

    A. mestranol
    B. clomiphene
    C. purified FSH
    D. topiramate
    E. bromocriptine

2. When assessing infertility, which of the following are important aspects of the male history? Select all that apply.

    A. occupation
    B. previous children
    C. sexual orientation
    D. frequency of intercourse
    E. religious beliefs

3. Which of the following are relative contraindications for the use of implantable contraceptives? Select all that apply.

    A. hypothyroidism
    B. history of asthma
    C. migraine headaches
    D. severe depression
    E. high cholesterol

CHAPTER 8

Genetics and Genetic Counseling

KEY TERMS

Please define the following terms:

Allele

Amniocentesis

Aneuploidy

Autosomes

Chromosome

Clastogen

Congenital

Cytogenetics

Deletion

Diploid

Dominant

Euploid

Gamete

Gametogenesis

Gene

Genetic counseling

Genetics

Genomics

Genotype

Haploid

Hemizygous

Heterozygote

Homologous

Homozygous

Karyotype

Maternal serum alpha-fetoprotein (MSAFP)

Meiosis

Mitosis

Monosomy

Mosaicism

Multifactorial

Mutation

Non-disjunction

Pedigree (genogram)

Personalized medicine

Phenotype

Polygenic

Proband

Recessive

Translocation

Trisomy

ACTIVITIES

1. List clastogens that can cause chromosome breakage.

2. What factors make chromosome breakage significant?

3. Identify and describe two types of translocation that have clinical significance.

4. Identify physiologic differences between oogenesis and spermatogenesis.

5. Distinguish the terms oogenesis and spermatogenesis.

6. Why aren't all women who are planning a pregnancy screened for genetic counseling?

7. Give an example of a continuous variation in a genetic trait.

8. List five diseases that are polygenic and multifactorial.

9. Summarize the characteristics of Ehlers-Danlos syndrome. How does this genetic disease complicate pregnancy?

10. List common physical alterations associated with Marfan syndrome.

11. Identify the complications of neurofibromatosis.

12. What are the characteristics of type I osteogenesis imperfecta?

13. Discuss the prognosis of a child with cystic fibrosis.

14. Explain the characteristics and complications of cystic fibrosis.

15. Discuss the complications of cystic fibrosis that may occur when a woman is pregnant.

16. Classify the types of mucopolysaccharidosis disorders.

17. Discuss the treatment for a woman with phenylketonuria (PKU).

18. Propose an educational plan for a woman diagnosed with PKU who is planning a pregnancy.

19. Explain the disease process of a client with sickle cell disease.

20. List common substances that may trigger glucose-6-phosphate dehydrogenase (G6PD) deficiency.

21. List the purposes for genetic screening.

22. When is screening for genetic disorders indicated?

23. Discuss the nursing role in genetic diagnostic testing and counseling.

24. Complete the following table for autosomal dominant disorders:

Disease	Characteristics	Effects on Pregnancy
Achondroplasia		
Ehlers-Danlos syndrome		
Marfan syndrome		
Neurofibromatosis (Type 1)		
Polycystic kidney disease		

25. Complete the following table for autosomal recessive disorders:

Disease	Characteristics	Effects on Pregnancy
Cystic fibrosis		
Mucopolysaccharidosis		
Phenylketonuria		
Sickle cell disease		
Tay-Sachs disease		

26. Complete the following table for X-linked disorders:

Disease	Characteristics	Effects on Pregnancy
Duchenne muscular dystrophy		
Glucose-6-phosphate dehydrogenase deficiency		
Hemophilia		

SELF-ASSESSMENT QUIZ

1. What hormone from the Leydig cells initiates spermatogenesis?

2. What is the most significant complication of Marfan syndrome?

3. When does polycystic kidney disease usually manifest itself?

4. Which type of mucopolysaccharidosis is the most common?

5. True or False

    T   F   Screening newborns for PKU is a legal requirement in all states.

    T   F   Infants born to mothers with treated PKU are not at risk for complications.

    T   F   Infants born with Tay-Sachs disease usually have a poor prognosis.

    T   F   Type III is the most common type of mucopolysaccharidosis.

6. Match the following genetic abnormality with the syndrome that it causes:

    _____ Trisomy 21   A. Patau syndrome

    _____ Trisomy 13–15   B. Klinefelter syndrome

    _____ Trisomy 18   C. Jacob's syndrome

    _____ XXY   D. Down syndrome

    _____ XYY   E. Edwards' syndrome

7. What substances may trigger hemolytic episodes in G6PD deficiency?

CRITICAL THINKING

Genetic screening is becoming more readily available all the time, and there are certainly many reasons for wanting to be tested. For example, if a woman discovered she carried a gene for breast cancer, she might be able to take steps to decrease her risk factors. Genetic testing may allow a woman to make informed reproductive choices. Most of us would agree to be tested when the knowledge gained could positively impact our future in some way.

Well, what if you were to find out that you carry the gene for a devastating disease, which will slowly rob you of your ability to function on any level? Furthermore, you discover that this illness will strike in the prime of your life, and currently, there is no treatment available. The disease is Huntington's chorea, or Huntington's disease.

Huntington's disease is an inherited, degenerative disorder of the central nervous system caused by a dominant gene. This means that everyone who inherits the gene will develop the disease.

Huntington's disease is basically a movement disorder. The earliest symptom is usually a sense of "clumsiness," eventually progressing to uncontrollable, bizarre movements. Other symptoms will include forgetfulness, irritability, and memory loss, eventually progressing to a severe form of dementia. The illness may continue relentlessly for 10–20 years once it has been diagnosed. Although research is underway, there is little hope for people suffering from this devastating disease. There are some medical ethicists that believe this kind of information should be withheld from afflicted individuals.

1. What is your opinion on telling people they have an incurable, fatal disease?

2. Would you want to know if you carried the gene for Huntington's disease?

3. What would you do with your life if you found out you had Huntington's disease?

4. Discuss the pros and cons of telling clients they have a disease such as Huntington's disease.

MULTIPLE CHOICE

1. Which of the following is a true statement regarding oogenesis?

   A. Oogenesis begins during puberty.
   B. Only about 50,000 eggs will reach full maturity.
   C. The process of oogenesis comprises four main phases.
   D. Long-term exposure of ova to environmental stimulants may correlate maternal age with birth defects.

2. A gene that determines a specific trait is called a(n) _____.

    A. phenotype
    B. allele
    C. genotype
    D. chromosome

3. Which of the following is a genetic disorder caused by a sex chromosome aneuploidy?

    A. Klinefelter syndrome
    B. neurofibromatosis
    C. Duchenne muscular dystrophy
    D. hemophilia

4. Which of the following disorders is characterized by scoliosis, tall stature, and the risk of a dissecting aortic aneurism?

    A. neurofibromatosis
    B. Ehlers-Danlos syndrome
    C. Turner syndrome
    D. Marfan syndrome

5. The study of chromosome abnormalities and Mendelian disorders is known as _____.

    A. genomics
    B. cytogenetics
    C. personalized medicine
    D. multifactorial inheritance

MULTIPLE RESPONSE

1. Which of the following are characteristics of dominant inheritance in an autosomal dominant pattern? Select all that apply.

    A. Children of the affected parent have a 75 percent chance of being affected.
    B. A carrier state does not exist.
    C. Females are more likely to be affected than males.
    D. The phenotype appears to skip generations.
    E. The homozygote for the mutant allele is likely to be more severely affected.

2. Which of the following are reasons for genetic screening? Select all that apply.

    A. to recognize a disease and provide early intervention
    B. to collect population data about a disease
    C. to provide a baseline of assessment data for current research studies
    D. to identify disease carriers and maximize parenthood options
    E. to disclose genetic risks to insurance carriers

3. Which of the following are true statements regarding Trisomy 18? Select all that apply.

    A. It may also be referred to as Patau syndrome.
    B. It is the most common genetic cause of severe learning disabilities in children.
    C. It may cause craniofacial, skeletal, cardiac, and urogenital abnormalities.
    D. It affects females more often than males.
    E. It leads to death in 30 percent of cases within the first month.

UNIT 4
Pregnancy

CHAPTER 9

Normal Pregnancy

KEY TERMS

Please define the following terms:

Amenorrhea

Ballottement

Braxton Hicks contractions

Chadwick's sign

Chloasma

Couvade

Goodell's sign

Hegar's sign

Hyperemesis gravidarum

Linea nigra

Physiologic anemia of pregnancy

Quickening

Striae gravidarum

Supine hypotension

ACTIVITIES

1. Are over-the-counter pregnancy tests accurate? How early can they detect pregnancy? What is the most common cause of false results?

2. Classify the following signs and symptoms according to presumptive, probable, and positive signs of pregnancy:

	Presumptive	Probable	Positive
Uterine enlargement			
Breast tenderness			
Quickening			
Urinary frequency			
Fetal heart sounds			
Goodell's sign			
Pregnancy test			
Visible fetus on ultrasound			

Chadwick's sign

Nausea or vomiting

_____

3. Calculate the following expected dates of delivery (EDD):

First Day of Last Menstrual Period	EDD
7/26/2012	
6/6/2013	
12/17/2013	
2/27/2012	

4. List physiologic changes due to pregnancy for the following body systems:

Body System or Organ	Expected Changes
Reproductive	
Breasts	
Cardiovascular	
Respiratory	
Gastrointestinal	
Endocrine	
Metabolic	
Urinary	

Integumentary

Musculoskeletal

---

5. Discuss the hematologic changes during pregnancy:

Constituent	Change
Plasma volume	
Total volume	
Hematocrit	
Hemoglobin	
Fibrinogen	
White blood cells	

---

6. Describe the process that leads to physiologic anemia of pregnancy.

7. What are the actions of the following hormones?
   Estrogen

   Progesterone

   Human chorionic gonadotropin

   Human placental lactogen

8. List the causes of water retention during pregnancy.

9. Differentiate the signs and symptoms of false labor and true labor.

10. What are the weight gain parameters for pregnant women who are normal weight, underweight, and obese at the onset of pregnancy?

11. Propose a client education plan for a woman with common complaints of pregnancy:

    Nausea or vomiting

    Heartburn

    Constipation

    Fatigue

    Urinary frequency

    Epistaxis or nasal congestion

    Varicosities

    Hemorrhoids

    Low back pain

    Leg cramps

12. Describe the impact smoking has on the fetus.

13. Discuss the impact pregnancy has on women in relation to the following:
    Workplace travel

    Lifestyle habits

    Acceptance of pregnancy

    Reflection

    Body image changes

14. Describe the role, changes, and cultural variations pregnancy has on the following groups:

Role	Changes	Cultural Variations
Maternal role		
Fatherhood		
Family unit		
Siblings		
Grandparents		

15. List nursing diagnoses from the North American Nursing Diagnosis Association that may be appropriate during pregnancy.

SELF-ASSESSMENT QUIZ

1. Match the term with the usual date it can be identified during pregnancy.

   _____ Quickening   A. 4 weeks

   _____ Fetal heartbeat by Doppler   B. 10–12 weeks

   _____ Ultrasound heartbeat   C. 18–20 weeks

2. True or False

   T   F   A systolic heart murmur is normal during pregnancy.

   T   F   Blood pressure always rises during the first trimester of pregnancy.

   T   F   The respiratory tidal volume decreases during pregnancy.

   T   F   Gingivitis is a common complication of pregnancy.

   T   F   Cavities are a common complication of pregnancy.

   T   F   Constipation is unusual during pregnancy.

3. What weight gain would you expect for a pregnant woman who is five feet, four inches tall and weighed 130 pounds prior to pregnancy?

4. A pregnant client tells you she is having constipation. She asks if she can take over-the-counter laxatives. How do you respond?

5. List three areas for health promotion for a pregnant woman.

CRITICAL THINKING

1. Describe the physiologic changes that occur during pregnancy that place a client at risk for gestational diabetes.

2. Mrs. Luna has just arrived at the midwife's office for a routine prenatal visit, and you will assist in determining maternal and fetal well-being.

   a. Mrs. Luna reports the first day of her last period was May 1. What would her expected due date be?

b. Based on Naegele's rule, you determine that Mrs. Luna is about 20 weeks' pregnant. Describe approximately where you should be able to palpate her fundus.

c. Mrs. Luna thinks she has been feeling her baby move. At what point in the pregnancy would you expect the mother to be able to feel movement?

d. Mrs. Luna tells you her gums have been bleeding lately when she brushes her teeth and wants to know why this is happening. How would you respond?

e. Mrs. Luna is planning on taking a long trip via automobile in one month. She is concerned about whether or not she should wear seatbelts. How would you respond?

f. Mrs. Luna is worried about getting stretch marks. She asks your advice about a cream she found in the back of a women's magazine that claims to prevent stretch marks. According to Mrs. Luna, her girlfriend used this product and did not get any marks on her abdomen. She wants your opinion and advice on preventing stretch marks. How would you respond?

MULTIPLE CHOICE

1. Which of the following hormones works to increase the capacity of the ureters and bladder during pregnancy?

   A. estrogen
   B. progesterone
   C. human chorionic gonadotropin
   D. human placental lactogen

2. Which of the following occurs as a change in the gastrointestinal system during pregnancy?

   A. There is a higher incidence of tooth loss.
   B. Blood flow to the liver is markedly changed, increasing the potential for hepatomegaly.
   C. The slow progression of the intestinal contents reduces absorption of nutrients.
   D. The effect of progesterone may result in an increased risk for gallstone formation.

3. A hormone secreted by the adrenal gland that promotes the metabolism of carbohydrates, protein, and fat is known as _____.

   A. cortisol
   B. angiotensin II
   C. renin
   D. aldosterone

4. Which of the following can be a sign of diabetic ketoacidosis during pregnancy?

    A. elevated blood glucose levels <100
    B. polydipsia and polyuria
    C. high blood pressure
    D. one plus pitting edema

5. Which of the following can the nurse recommend to the pregnant client suffering from back pain?

    A. Keep the back straight with the pelvis tilted backward.
    B. Practice deep breathing exercises that focus directly on the pain.
    C. Wear comfortable, low-heeled shoes.
    D. Increase sleep by three hours each night.

MULTIPLE RESPONSE

1. Which of the following is a role of estrogen during pregnancy? Select all that apply.

    A. relaxing smooth muscles of the gastrointestinal tract to improve nutrient absorption
    B. softening the cervix in preparation for labor
    C. suppressing the immunologic response of the maternal body to the fetus
    D. increasing blood flow to the uterus by promoting vasodilation
    E. developing the breasts in preparation for lactation

2. Which of the following are signs of true labor? Select all that apply.

    A. Pain begins in the abdomen and moves toward the lower back.
    B. The cervix is firm and feels similar to the top of the ear.
    C. Bloody show from the vagina is present and is pinkish or blood-streaked.
    D. Contractions intensify and do not ease, despite activity.
    E. Contractions become more frequent, regular, and painful.

3. Which of the following occurs as a change in the hematologic system during pregnancy? Select all that apply.

    A. Hematocrit levels decrease.
    B. Hemoglobin levels decrease.
    C. Plasma volumes increase.
    D. Fibrinogen levels decrease.
    E. Blood leukocyte counts decrease.

CHAPTER 10

Nursing Care of the Pregnant Woman

KEY TERMS

Please define the following terms:

Bi-ischial diameter

Childbirth education

Cleansing breath

Doula

Estimated date of birth (EDB)

Estimated date of confinement (EDC)

Estimated due date (EDD)

Fetal alcohol syndrome (FAS)

Fetal movement count (FMC)

Gestational hypertension

Gravida

Gravida, term, para, abortion, living (GTPAL)

Health maintenance

Health promotion

Hyperemesis gravidarum

Interspinous diameter

Intrauterine growth restriction (IUGR)

Last menstrual period (LMP)

Macrosomia

Midpelvis

Montrice

Multigravida

Multipara

Naegele's Rule

Obstetrical conjugate

Paced breathing

Para

Pelvic inlet

Pelvic outlet

Perinatal education

Pica

Preconception care

Pre-eclampsia

Prenatal care

Primigravida

Primipara

Quickening

Teratogen

ACTIVITIES

1. As a nurse, how can you help clients overcome barriers to prenatal care?

2. List diagnostic tests to be done at the first prenatal visit.

3. What is the current recommendation for folic acid supplementation for a woman during pregnancy?

4. Determine whether the following diagnostic tests are done on the initial visit, all visits, or at specific intervals. Place a check mark in the appropriate column:

Diagnostic Test or Assessment	Initial Visit	All Visits	Specific Time Interval
Blood pressure			
Urinalysis			
Complete blood count			
Facial edema			
Fetal heart tones			
Rh factor			
Blood type			
Cervical and vaginal cultures			
Fundal height			
Alpha-fetoprotein			
Edema of lower extremities			
Hemoglobin and Hematocrit			

Group B streptococci

Cervical dilation

---

5. Determine when the following discomforts of pregnancy are most likely to occur. List the causes and possible complications, and then develop interventions:

Discomfort	Cause	Complications	Interventions
Urinary frequency			
Nausea or vomiting			
Indigestion			
Constipation			
Hemorrhoids			
Edema of lower extremities			

6. Propose an educational plan to teach a client the danger signs that must be evaluated.

7. List and discuss which pregnant women are considered to be at increased risk for vitamin and mineral deficiencies.

SELF-ASSESSMENT QUIZ

1. What immunizations are contraindicated during pregnancy?

2. True or False

    T F Edema of the face and hands is expected in the last trimester of pregnancy.

    T F The location of a prenatal clinic can be a barrier to accessing care for many women.

T   F   Prenatal education should start with the last trimester of pregnancy.

T   F   Pregnancy confirmation is a primary cause for clients to seek medical attention.

T   F   It is recommended that an overweight woman diet during pregnancy.

T   F   The U.S. Food and Drug Administration recommends that pregnant women eliminate dietary caffeine.

T   F   Pica is the persistent ingestion of non-nutritive substances.

3. Determine whether the following are common discomforts (A) or danger signs (B) of pregnancy.

_____ Vaginal bleeding

_____ Indigestion

_____ Urinary frequency

_____ Swelling of feet

_____ Swelling of face and hands

_____ Abdominal pain

_____ Nausea

_____ Severe headache

_____ Vomiting

_____ Sudden gush of vaginal fluid

_____ Constipation

4. A woman who has twins who are four years old, a baby who is two years old, and is now pregnant is gravida _____, para _____.

CRITICAL THINKING

1. The registered nurse is required to perform phone triage for the health department. A client calls and reports the following: "I am six and a half months pregnant, and this is my second baby. I have been feeling OK until last night, when I began having pain in my back. What should I do?"

   a. What probable reasons could there be for this client to have back pain?

   b. What further questions would you ask her to determine the cause of the back pain?

   c. The client describes her pain as constant and burning. She reports dysuria, urinary frequency, and some shaking chills. How would you respond at this time?

2. When a woman is pregnant, well-meaning people often feel it is necessary to provide unsolicited advice and suggestions. Often their words of wisdom are based on old wives' tales and not science. Just for fun, read the following list of old wives' tales and see if you have heard of them and can add to the list.

   ■ Looking at a rabbit while pregnant will cause the baby to be born with a harelip.

   ■ Eating strawberries will cause the baby to be born with a strawberry mark on the skin.

   ■ If the woman is carrying larger in the front, the baby will be a boy. If the woman is carrying larger in the back, the baby will be a girl.

   ■ Stretch marks are caused by not drinking enough milk.

   ■ Keeping a knife under the mattress of a laboring woman will cut the pain of labor.

   ■ Wearing red will protect the pregnant woman and her baby from evil wishes.

   ■ More women go into labor during a full moon.

MULTIPLE CHOICE

1. A client is seen for her first prenatal visit. The first day of her LMP was September 8. According to Naegele's Rule, this client would have an EDC of _____.

   A. July 1
   B. July 15

   C. May 30
   D. June 15

2. The pelvis is visually divided into three planes during assessment. The first plane is the _____.

   A. obstetrical conjugate
   B. pelvic inlet
   C. interpelvis
   D. interspinous diameter

3. A method of childbirth preparation that focuses on a totally natural birthing process and emphasizes the importance of the partner in the coaching role is called the _____.

   A. Lamaze method
   B. relaxation method
   C. Bradley method
   D. Dick-Read method

4. A nurse who can provide nursing care and assessment in addition to labor support is known as a _____.

   A. montrice
   B. doula
   C. midwife
   D. childbirth educator

5. A labor technique that focuses on differentiating relaxation from tension is known as _____.

   A. imagery
   B. effleurage
   C. slow-paced breathing
   D. neuromuscular dissociation

MULTIPLE RESPONSE

1. Which of the following instructions should the nurse give to the pregnant client in order to perform fetal movement counts? Select all that apply.

   A. The best time to count fetal movements is right after waking up in the morning.
   B. Understand that the fetus will have periods of activity and periods of sleeping.
   C. Count every five feelings of motion from the fetus as one movement.
   D. Sit comfortably in a quiet place to pay attention to fetal movements.
   E. Call the health care provider if the baby has not moved all day.

2. Which of the following guidelines can the nurse give to the pregnant client to reduce the risk of toxoplasmosis? Select all that apply.

   A. Use work gloves when gardening and wash your hands afterward.
   B. Do not allow your cat to come indoors.
   C. Cover children's sandboxes when not in use.
   D. Avoid eating raw fruits and vegetables.
   E. Wash your hands thoroughly after preparing raw meat.

3. A client presents for prenatal care at 10 weeks' gestation. Which of the following are laboratory tests to be completed at the initial prenatal visit? Select all that apply.

   A. glucose screening
   B. urinalysis
   C. hematocrit
   D. hepatitis screen
   E. AFP screening

CHAPTER 11

Management and Nursing Care of High-Risk Clients

KEY TERMS

Please define the following terms:

ABO incompatibility

Abortion

Abruptio placentae

Acquired immunodeficiency syndrome (AIDS)

Adolescence

Adolescent pregnancy

Amniocentesis

Antiretroviral therapy

Cerclage

Chronic hypertension

Cognitive development

Developmental tasks

Disseminated intravascular coagulation (DIC)

Dizygotic

Eclampsia

Ectopic pregnancy

Elective abortion

Gestational diabetes

Gestational trophoblastic disease

Human immunodeficiency virus (HIV)

Hydramnios

Hydrops fetalis

Incompetent cervix

Induced abortion

Ketoacidosis

Macrosomia

Marginal placenta previa

Monozygotic

Oligohydramnios

Partial previa

Percutaneous umbilical blood sampling (PUBS)

Placenta previa

Polyhydramnios

Postterm pregnancy

Pre-eclampsia

Premature rupture of membranes (PROM)

Preterm labor

Preterm premature rupture of membranes (PPROM)

Seroconversion

Sexual maturation

Spontaneous abortion

Therapeutic abortion

Thrombocytopenia

Thyrotoxicosis

Type I diabetes mellitus

Type II diabetes mellitus

Vertical transmission

ACTIVITIES

1. Categorize various types of spontaneous abortions.

2. List the signs and symptoms of a threatening abortion.

3. Discuss the medical and nursing management of a client with an ectopic pregnancy.

4. Describe the following placental abnormalities.
   Placenta previa

   Marginal placenta previa

Low-lying placenta

Abruptio placentae

5. Discuss the incidence, clinical presentation, and medical and nursing management of placental abnormalities.

6. Define disseminated intravascular coagulation (DIC). Which clients are at increased risk for DIC?

7. Discuss the clinical presentation, treatment, and teaching of the following labor disorders:

Disorder	Clinical Presentation	Treatment	Teaching
Incompetent cervix			
Preterm labor			
Premature rupture of membranes			
Preterm premature rupture of membranes			
Postterm pregnancy			

8. Describe the indications, side effects, and complications of the following drugs used during labor and delivery:

Drug	Indications	Side Effects	Complications
Magnesium sulfate			
Beta-adrenergics			
Prostaglandin inhibitors			
Calcium channel blockers			

9. Discuss the complications that may occur with polyhydramnios.

10. List the possible causes of oligohydramnios.

11. What maternal and fetal effects may multiple gestations have?

12. Discuss Rh isoimmunization and ABO incompatibility.

13. Discuss the pharmacotherapeutics of RhoGam.

14. Explain the definition, classification, pathophysiology, and management of hypertensive disorders of pregnancy.

15. Recall the effects of hypertension on the following systems and the fetus:
Cardiopulmonary

Renal

Neurologic

Hematologic

Hepatic

Fetus

16. Differentiate the three categories of diabetes.

    Type I

    Type II

    Gestational

17. Describe the diagnostic criteria for the three-hour glucose tolerance test for gestational diabetes.

18. Propose a client education plan for a woman with gestational diabetes.

19. Compare hypothyroidism and hyperthyroidism.

Disorder	Diagnosis	Clinical Manifestations	Medical Management	Nursing Care	Effects on Fetus
Hypothyroidism					
Hyperthyroidism					

20. Discuss cardiovascular disorders that place the mother and fetus at risk during pregnancy and delivery.

21. Complete the table on disorders that may affect or can be affected by pregnancy.

Disorder	Description	Clinical Presentation	Medical Management	Nursing Care	Effects on Fetus
Asthma					
Tuberculosis					

Thrombocytopenic purpura

Sickle cell disease

Seizure disorders

---

22. What are the possible side effects of anticonvulsant medications?

23. Discuss medical and nursing management of the pregnant client infected with HIV.

24. List the means of transmission of HIV from a mother to her baby.

25. How does the United States compares to other developed countries in relation to adolescent pregnancy?

26. Identify factors that contribute to the decline of adolescent pregnancy in the United States.

27. Compare factors that contribute to adolescent pregnancy for various populations.

Adolescents in General	Affluent Adolescents	Poor Adolescents

28. Discuss the effects of adolescent pregnancy on psychosocial development.

Theory	Task	Description	Effect	Nursing Implications
Erikson				
Piaget				

29. Complete the following table:

	Early Adolescence	Middle Adolescence	Late Adolescence
Cognitive thinking	1.	1.	1.
	2.	2.	2.
	3.	3.	3.
Issues in sexuality	1.	1.	1.
	2.	2.	2.
	3.	3.	3.
Issues in pregnancy	1.	1.	1.
	2.	2.	2.
	3.	3.	3.

30. Discuss factors that contribute to adolescent pregnancy.

31. Using a lab partner, perform an assessment of sexual history for an adolescent.

32. Discuss nursing interventions for obstetric complications for a pregnant adolescent.

Complication	Nursing Interventions
Poor nutrition	
Pregnancy-induced hypertension	

33. Identify women at risk for HIV or AIDS.

34. Discuss pre- and post-test counseling for clients with HIV or AIDS.

35. Describe opportunistic infections that infants with HIV are likely to manifest.

36. List the common side effects of zidovudine therapy.

SELF-ASSESSMENT QUIZ

1. What is the most common cause of disseminated intravascular coagulation (DIC)?

2. True or False

   T   F   In the majority of cases of severe polyhydramnios, a fetal anomaly is present.

   T   F   Oligohydramnios usually develops in early pregnancy.

   T   F   If the mother is Rh positive and the fetus is Rh negative, RhoGam is indicated.

   T   F   Hypertension is defined as a blood pressure ≥ 140 mmHg systolic or ≥ 90 mmHg diastolic.

T   F   Adolescent minority males are more likely than adolescent minority females to contract AIDS.

T   F   AIDS is the third leading cause of death for all women ages 25–34.

T   F   In uninfected neonates, the maternal HIV antibodies will disappear by approximately 18 months of age.

T   F   Opportunistic infections and clinical symptoms of AIDS usually occur when the CD4+T-lymphocyte cell count declines.

3. The Rh-negative mother of an Rh-positive infant should receive prophylaxis RhoGam within _____ hours.

4. List the indications for insulin therapy for gestational diabetes.

5. List five factors that contribute to adolescent pregnancy.

6. Who has the greatest risk for obstetric complications?

7. What are three ways HIV can be transferred from mother to baby?

8. List five areas of prenatal education for the adolescent mother.

CRITICAL THINKING

Sara presents at the E.R. with complaints of vaginal bleeding, lower abdominal pain, and syncope. Her last menstrual period was six weeks ago. Her blood pressure is 100/50 mmHg, and pulse is 120 bpm. Her history is significant due to an episode of pelvic inflammatory disease three years ago and treatment for a chlamydia infection.

1. What symptoms made the health care team suspicious of an ectopic pregnancy?

2. What factor(s) place Sara at risk for an ectopic pregnancy?

3. What is the greatest medical risk to Sara at this time?

4. What diagnostic study is used to identify an ectopic pregnancy?

MULTIPLE CHOICE

1. Which of the following is a potential side effect following the administration of magnesium sulfate in managing pre-eclampsia?

    A. hyperglycemia
    B. pulmonary edema
    C. gastrointestinal bleeding
    D. hypokalemia

2. Hypertension that occurs before pregnancy or is diagnosed before 20 weeks' gestation is called _____.

    A. chronic hypertension
    B. pre-eclampsia
    C. eclampsia
    D. gestational hypertension

3. Which of the following is an adverse outcome associated with hyperthyroidism?

    A. cretinism
    B. respiratory arrest
    C. seizures
    D. congestive heart failure

4. Which test initially confirms HIV seroconversion in a pregnant woman?

    A. western blot
    B. immunoglobulin G (IgG)
    C. ELISA
    D. polymerase chain reaction (PCR)

5. Which of the following is a sexuality issue for an early adolescent who engages in concrete thinking?

    A. changing body image
    B. responsible sexual decision making
    C. correct use of contraception
    D. set sexual preferences

MULTIPLE RESPONSE

1. Which of the following have been implicated as possible causes of ectopic pregnancy? Select all that apply.

    A. chromosomal abnormalities of the embryo
    B. multiple induced abortions
    C. peritoneal dialysis
    D. previous use of methotrexate
    E. history of placenta previa

2. Which of the following are nursing care measures for the client with gestational trophoblastic disease? Select all that apply.

    A. Assess vaginal bleeding.
    B. Record urinary output.
    C. Perform skin assessments.
    D. Palpate fundal height.
    E. Educate the client regarding contraception.

3. Which of the following are potential complications to the fetus related to pregnancy-induced hypertension? Select all that apply.

    A. cephalhematoma
    B. high blood pressure
    C. prematurity
    D. intrauterine growth restriction
    E. hypoxia

CHAPTER 12

Fetal Development

KEY TERMS

Please define the following terms:

Amnion

Amniotic fluid

Blastocyst

Chorion

Chorionic villi

Decidua

Decidua basalis

Decidua capsularis

Decidua parietalis

Embryo

Fertilization

Fetal alcohol spectrum disorders

Heavy metal

Herbicide

Human chorionic gonadotropin (hCG)

Human placental lactogen (hPL)

Hyperthermia

Implantation

Lanugo

Meiosis

Mitosis

Morula

Neonatal abstinence syndrome

Pesticide

Spermatozoa

Teratogen

TORCH

Trophoblast cells

Wharton's jelly

Zygote

ACTIVITIES

1. Describe the travel of the zygote from the fallopian tube to implantation in the endometrium.

2. Explain problems that could occur with low implantation of the zygote in the endometrium.

3. Discuss the probability of the proper implantation of a zygote that will progress to pregnancy.

4. Describe the three regions of the decidua.

5. Summarize the growth and development of the placenta from implantation to term.

6. Describe the two parts of the placenta: maternal and fetal.

7. Define the metabolic functions of the placenta.

8. Describe the endocrine function in pregnancy.

9. Describe the function of progesterone in pregnancy.

10. Describe placental circulation.

11. Differentiate between fetal and newborn circulation. Identify the functions of the foramen ovale, the ductus venosus, and the ductus arteriosus.

12. Identify the function of the umbilical cord.

13. Define the function of Wharton's jelly.

14. Explain the functions of the amnion and the chorion.

15. Describe the composition and function of amniotic fluid.

16. Define the embryonic stage.

17. Describe the embryonic disc at three weeks' gestation.

18. Propose a client education plan to help reduce the risks to a pregnant woman in the workforce.

19. What preconceptual counseling information should a nurse provide to a woman on medications for a chronic disease?

20. List the five categories the U.S. Food and Drug Administration (FDA) uses to classify drugs according to their risk in pregnancy.

21. While performing client education for a pregnant woman, what medicines can the nurse recommend for common complaints?

22. Why should women avoid alcohol use during pregnancy?

23. Discuss the signs and symptoms of fetal alcohol spectrum disorders.

24. How does nicotine affect a fetus?

25. Complete the following table on illicit drug use during pregnancy:

Illicit Drug	Effect on Pregnancy and Fetus
Marijuana	
Cocaine	
Heroin	

26. Other than the effects of the drug itself, what complications does illicit drug use have on the pregnant woman and the fetus?

27. How do sexually transmitted diseases (STDs) affect pregnancy and the fetus?

STD	Effect on Pregnant Woman	Effect on Fetus or Newborn	Nursing Intervention
Syphilis			
Gonorrhea			
Chlamydia			
Herpes simplex virus			
Human immunodeficiency virus			

28. Complete the following table on infectious diseases and their effects on pregnancy:

Infection	Effect on Woman	Effect on Fetus or Newborn	Nursing Intervention
Hepatitis B			
Varicella-zoster virus (chickenpox)			
Cytomegalovirus			
Toxoplasmosis			
Streptococcus			
Rubella			

29. List the routine assessment of fetal well-being.

30. List nursing diagnoses, causes, and potential outcomes for pregnant clients with infections.

31. Describe important points to remember when asking the pregnant client about substance abuse.

32. Discuss potential risks to the fetus that a pregnant client may encounter in the environment, at work, and in the home.

33. Name several guidelines that a pregnant client can follow to reduce the risks of work in pregnancy.

34. Explain standard precautions to prevent the spread of infection.

35. Describe the TORCH screen and its components.

SELF-ASSESSMENT QUIZ

1. Differentiate between mitosis and meiosis.

2. The mature ovum and sperm each have _____ chromosomes.

3. True or False

   T   F   Fertilization occurs within 24 to 48 hours after release of the ovum into the uterus.

   T   F   The fertilized ovum forms the fetus and the accessory structures needed to support intrauterine life.

   T   F   The placenta eventually serves as the lungs, kidneys, endocrine system, and gastrointestinal tract for the fetus.

   T   F   The fetal portion of the placenta is red, rough, and segmented.

   T   F   Maternal blood mixes with fetal blood in the placenta.

T   F   By the seventh week the placenta produces more than 50% of the estrogen in the maternal circulation.

T   F   The two umbilical arteries carry oxygenated blood to the fetus, and the vein carries deoxygenated blood away from the fetus.

4. Every organ and external structure found in the full-term newborn is present at what week of embryonic development?

5. After the eighth week, the remainder of gestation is devoted to what development?

6. Match the following gestational stages with their description.

_____ Embryonic stage   A. The cardiovascular system begins to form, and blood begins to circulate within the premature heart.

_____ 3 weeks   B. Partitioning of the heart occurs with the dividing of the atrium.

_____ 4 weeks   C. The beginnings of all essential external and internal structures are present.

_____ 5 weeks   D. The circulatory system is well established through the umbilical cord.

_____ 6 weeks   E. The forming of external features and essential organs.

_____ 7 weeks   F. If the fetus is male, the testes begin to descend into the scrotal sac.

_____ 8 weeks   G. Main divisions of the central nervous system are established.

_____ 9–12 weeks   H. The liver starts to produce blood cells.

_____ 13–16 weeks   I. The fetus has nails on fingers and toes.

_____ 17–19 weeks   J. Bones are now fully developed, but are soft and flexible.

_____ 20–23 weeks   K. The body and extremities are plump with good skin turgor.

_____ 24 weeks   L. Fetal heart tones may be heard through a stethoscope.

_____ 25–28 weeks   M. Tooth buds appear for all 20 of the child's first teeth.

_____ 29–32 weeks   N. Skin ridges on the palms and soles form distinct finger-prints and footprints.

_____ 33–36 weeks   O. Fetus has a firm grasp.

_____ 38–40 weeks   P. Liver and pancreas begin to function.

7. What is the FDA category for the following teratogenic risks?

_____ Studies in animals or humans have demonstrated fetal abnormalities.

_____ Controlled studies in women fail to demonstrate a risk to the fetus in the first trimester or later trimesters.

_____ Animal reproduction studies have not demonstrated a fetal risk, but no controlled studies in pregnant women are available.

_____ Studies in animals have revealed adverse effects on the fetus, and there are no controlled studies in women.

_____ There is positive evidence of human fetal risk, but benefits from use may be acceptable despite the risk.

8. What is the leading cause of childhood mental retardation?

9. What does the acronym TORCH stand for?

10. Match the following terms with their definition.

_____ Ductus arteriosus   A. Opening between right and left atria

_____ Ductus venousus   B. Carries oxygenated blood from placenta to fetus

_____ Foramen ovale   C. Fetal blood vessel that allows blood to bypass liver

_____ Umbilical vein   D. Fetal blood vessel connecting the pulmonary artery to the aorta

11. Identify three disciplines that are included in fetal evaluation.

12. What is the average duration of human pregnancy?

CRITICAL THINKING

1. You are the triage nurse working in a women's health clinic. Susan J. is a 15-year-old girl who arrives in the clinic with complaints of vaginal itching and a foul odor coming from her vaginal area. She is diagnosed with chlamydia, but Susan denies having had sexual relations. How would you manage this?

MULTIPLE CHOICE

1. The inner membrane that surrounds the fetus and begins to develop in the second week of gestation is called the _____.

   A. chorion
   B. amnion

   C. Wharton's jelly
   D. amniotic fluid

2. The fetal shunt that connects the pulmonary artery to the descending aorta and that closes after birth is called the _____.

   A. foramen ovale
   B. ductus arteriosus

   C. umbilical cord
   D. ductus venosus

3. Which of the following illnesses causes limb hypoplasia, eye anomalies, and mental retardation of the fetus if infection occurs during the first trimester of pregnancy?

   A. toxoplasmosis
   B. cytomegalovirus

   C. varicella zoster
   D. hepatitis

4. The "H" portion of the TORCH screen stands for which infection?

   A. herpes simplex virus
   B. human immunodeficiency virus

   C. hantavirus
   D. hepadnovirus D

5. At what week of gestation does the fetus begin a regular schedule of sucking, kicking, and sleeping?

   A. week 12
   B. week 16

   C. week 20
   D. week 24

MULTIPLE RESPONSE

1. Which of the following occur at approximately six weeks' gestation? Select all that apply.

   A. The fetus resembles a human being.
   B. Primitive kidneys form.
   C. Tooth buds appear.
   D. Lung buds are present.
   E. Heart development is complete.

2. Which of the following drugs have been proven to be teratogens? Select all that apply.

   A. phenytoin
   B. methotrexate
   C. oral polio vaccine
   D. lithium
   E. acetaminophen

3. Which of the following statements are true about babies born to women who smoke during pregnancy? Select all that apply.

A. They have 75 percent higher odds of being born prematurely.
B. They are more likely to be born with low-birth weight.
C. They are up to three times more likely to die of SIDS.
D. They weigh approximately 200 grams less than babies born to women who do not smoke.
E. They have a 50 percent greater chance of being born with lung disease.

CHAPTER 13

Fetal Assessment

KEY TERMS

Please define the following terms:

Acceleration

Amniocentesis

Amnioinfusion

Biophysical profile (BPP)

Chorionic villus sampling (CVS)

Contraction stress test (CST)

Doppler blood studies

Fetal fibronectin (fFN) testing

Fetal movement counting (FMC)

Fetal tissue sampling

Human chorionic gonadotropin (hCG)

Human placental lactogen (hPL)

Inhibin-A

Magnetic resonance imaging (MRI)

Maternal serum alpha-fetoprotein (MS-AFP) testing

Non-stress test (NST)

Nuchal translucency

Percutaneous umbilical blood sampling (PUBS)

Ultrasonography

ACTIVITIES

1. Complete the table on fetal surveillance procedures:

	Diagnostic Testing	Screening Procedures	Reassurance Procedures
Test			
Definition			
When performed			
Expected outcomes			
Possible outcomes			
Nursing implications			

2. When should fetal surveillance procedures be considered for women?

3. What are the nursing responsibilities in fetal surveillance procedures?

4. Propose a client education plan for fetal evaluation procedures. Use the following client education questions:

   Why is the procedure being done?

   Is the procedure safe?

   Who will perform the procedure?

   How accurate is the test?

   What will the test tell us?

   Is any physical preparation necessary?

   What does the procedure involve?

   What will the client feel?

   How much time will the test take?

   What is the recovery time after the procedure?

   Who will interpret the results?

   When will the client be informed of the results?

   Who will talk with the client about the results?

What are the client's specific fears and concerns about the test?

What other options are available?

5. Differentiate between invasive diagnostic studies and maternal serum studies. Give examples of each.

6. List the indications for amniocentesis.

7. What information can the results of an amniocentesis provide?

8. A client tells you her primary care provider has recommended she have an amniocentesis. She asks you what the procedure is like. How will you answer her question?

9. Describe the nursing care provided after an amniocentesis. Include areas for client education.

10. What are the advantages and disadvantages of CVS?

11. List the genetic and biochemical conditions PUBS can diagnose.

12. List hormone levels that are included in maternal serum studies.

13. What defects does the MS-AFP test screen for?

14. Which clients should have the MS-AFP screening?

15. List factors that can affect the MS-AFP levels.

16. Complete the following table on MS-AFP testing:

Test	Possible Results	Outcomes	Implications	Complications
Estrogen				
Estriol				
Maternal serum alpha-fetoprotein				
Fetal cell isolation				
Human chorionic gonadotropin				

17. What information does an ultrasound provide about a fetus, the placenta, and the uterus?

18. When should an ultrasound be performed during pregnancy? What are the indications for an ultrasound?

19. Differentiate between abdominal ultrasound and transvaginal ultrasound.

20. Describe information provided by Doppler flow studies.

21. How can vibroacoustic stimulation help clarify a false positive NST?

22. Describe the procedure for a CST.

23. List factors that can influence fetal movement.

24. Propose an education plan to instruct a client in performing and documenting fetal movement counts.

25. Explain the scoring for a BPP.

26. When is a BPP indicated?

27. Differentiate various fetal surveillance tests by completing the following table:

Test	Abbreviation	When Performed	Client Preparation	Complications	Nursing Responsibilities
Amniocentesis					
Chorionic villus sampling					
Fetal tissue sampling					
Percutaneous umbilical blood sampling					
Fetal fibronectin					
Ultrasound					
Doppler blood studies					
Magnetic resonance imaging					
Fetal heart rate monitoring					
Non-stress testing					
Contraction stress test					
Fetal movement counts					

28. List nursing diagnoses from the North American Nursing Diagnosis Association that may be appropriate for clients during fetal evaluation testing.

29. Propose outcomes for the client undergoing fetal evaluation.

30. List three ethical issues and three legal issues that might result from fetal surveillance procedures.

SELF-ASSESSMENT QUIZ

1. List hormone levels that are included in maternal serum studies.

2. Match the results with the definition for a contraction stress test (CST).

_____ Late decelerations occur with less than half the uterine contractions.

A. Negative

_____ No late decelerations with three adequate uterine contractions in a 10-minute window, normal baseline fetal heart rate (FHR), and accelerations with fetal movement.

B. Positive

_____ Late decelerations occur with more than half the uterine contractions.

C. Suspicious

_____ Inadequate fetal heart rate (FHR) recording or less than three uterine contractions in 10 minutes.

D. Unsatisfactory

3. What surveillance technique is an accurate indication of impending fetal demise?

4. List the indications for non-stress testing.

CRITICAL THINKING CASE

Mrs. B. is a 37-year-old, G1P0 client who comes to the clinic for a regularly scheduled prenatal visit. She is 18 weeks pregnant and has been told that she had an abnormal result on her maternal serum alpha-fetoprotein (MS-AFP) test, which will need further evaluation. Mrs. B. has an aunt with Down syndrome and is aware of her own age as being a potential risk factor for genetic abnormalities for her baby. She is afraid of having a baby with Down syndrome and states that if she found out that this was the case, she is not sure that she could continue the pregnancy.

1. What are Mrs. B.'s risk factors for having a baby born with genetic abnormalities?

2. After an abnormal MS-AFP result, what is the next type of testing that may be performed in this situation?

3. How would the nurse explain upcoming procedures to this client in order to prepare her for the testing process?

4. Mrs. B. asks if the tests will hurt. How does the nurse respond?

5. What can the nurse do to help Mrs. B. as she manages conflicting feelings about the outcomes of this pregnancy?

MULTIPLE CHOICE

1. Which of the following questions should the nurse ask herself when considering whether prenatal screening should be done?

   A. Does insurance cover this procedure?
   B. What is the risk to the pregnancy?
   C. Do I know how to perform this procedure?
   D. Is there another method available?

2. Which of the following is a potential complication following amniocentesis?

   A. kidney pain
   B. bladder rupture

   C. yeast infection
   D. Rh isoimmunization

3. A direct biopsy of the fetus using biopsy forceps is called _____.

   A. fetal tissue sampling
   B. fetal fibronectin testing

   C. alpha-fetoprotein
   D. percutaneous umbilical blood sampling

4. Which of the following is an indication for a non-stress test?

   A. significant uterine size
   B. vaginal bleeding

   C. history of previous stillbirth
   D. evaluation of fetal growth

5. A gradual decrease in the fetal heart rate that is related to uterine contractions is known as a(n) _____.

   A. early deceleration
   B. late deceleration
   C. variable deceleration
   D. acceleration

MULTIPLE RESPONSE

1. Which of the following are components of the quad screen? Select all that apply.

   A. inhibin-A
   B. human chorionic gonadotropin (hCG)
   C. estrogen
   D. human placental lactogen (hPL)
   E. maternal serum alpha-fetoprotein (MS-AFP)

2. Which of the following are indications for amniocentesis during the first half of pregnancy? Select all that apply.

   A. Rh isoimmunization
   B. maternal age over 35 years
   C. family history of neural tube defect
   D. history of spontaneous abortion
   E. elevated MS-AFP level

3. Which of the following are types of fetal surveillance procedures that are considered reassurance measures? Select all that apply.

   A. biophysical profile (BPP)
   B. fetal movement counting (FMC)
   C. fetal fibronectin screening (fFN)
   D. non-stress test
   E. chorionic villus sampling

UNIT 5
Childbirth

CHAPTER 14

Processes of Labor and Delivery

KEY TERMS

Please define the following terms:

Active phase

Amniotomy

Augmentation of labor

Bloody show

Braxton Hicks contractions

Cervical dilation

Cesarean section

Crowning

Descent

Dystocia

Effacement

Engagement

False pelvis

Fetal attitude

Fetal lie

Fetal position

Fetal presentation

First stage of labor

Flexion

Fontanels

Forceps

Gap junctions

Interventions of labor

Labor

Labor induction

Latent phase

Leopold's maneuvers

Lightening

Maternal role attainment

Molding

Nesting

Oxytocin

Parturition

Placental stage

Primary powers

Pushing stage

Second stage of labor

Secondary powers

Station

Third stage of labor

Transition

ACTIVITIES

1. Describe each of the five Ps of the labor process.

   (1) Passageway

        True pelvis

        False pelvis

        Station

   (2) Passenger

        Fetal head size

        Fetal presentation

        Fetal lie

        Fetal attitude

        Fetal position

        Assessment of fetal presentation and position

        Leopold's four maneuvers or abdominal palpation

Vaginal examination

(3) Primary and secondary powers

(4) Position

(5) Psychologic response of the mother

Factors that make labor a meaningful, positive event

Cultural perceptions of childbirth

2. Define and compare the following signs and symptoms of impending labor:

Lightening

Cervical changes

Braxton Hicks contractions

Bloody show

Energy spurt

Nesting

Gastrointestinal disturbances

3. Describe and explain the stages of labor:

First stage

      Latent phase

      Active phase

      Transition phase

Second stage

      Pushing

      Crowning

      Cardinal movements or mechanisms of labor

      Descent

      Flexion

      Internal rotation

      Extension

      Restitution

      External rotation

      Expulsion

Third stage (placental stage)

Fourth stage (recovery stage)

4. Describe labor induction and the use of Bishop's scoring system.

5. Explain the advantages and disadvantages of several cervical ripening methods.

6. Differentiate among the different types of interventions of labor:
Labor induction

Cervical ripening method

Amniotomy

Augmentation of labor

Forceps-assisted birth

Vacuum-assisted birth

Cesarean birth

7. Explain the maternal physiologic adaptations to the process of labor that occur in each of the following systems:
Hematologic system

Cardiovascular system

Respiratory system

Renal system

Gastrointestinal system

Endocrine system

8. Describe the positions for fetal presentation:
   Vertex presentation

   Face presentation

   Breech presentation

9. Describe the presenting part of the fetus in relation to the four quadrants of the maternal pelvis.

10. Identify the various surgical incisions made in the mother for a cesarean section.

11. The fetal heart rate (FHR) can be auscultated in various areas. Identify these areas.

12. Explain the use of oxytocin in the birthing process.

SELF-ASSESSMENT QUIZ

1. Identify the process and time element associated with the four stages of labor:

Stage	Process	Time Element
1		
2		
3		
4		

2. If situations arise that do not allow a spontaneous vaginal delivery, what are the options available to the health care provider?

3. Name the five Ps that are important factors that affect the process of labor.

4. Differentiate between the false and true pelvis.

5. Differentiate between effacement and cervical dilation.

6. Compare molding and fontanels.

7. Compare primary and secondary powers.

CRITICAL THINKING

Mrs. M. is a gravida three, para two who is admitted to the nursing unit in early labor. The initial exam reveals her cervix is two cm dilated, 50% effaced, and -1 station. Her contractions are coming every ten to fifteen minutes and lasting 30–40 seconds. Seven hours later, your assessment reveals that her cervix is unchanged and her contractions are still only coming every seven to ten minutes and lasting 30–40 seconds. The midwife decides to start the client on oxytocin.

1. What is the average length of time for the latent phase to last for a multigravida?

2. What would a safe starting dose of oxytocin be for this client?

3. What are the three purposes of an oxytocin administration?

4. What are the priority nursing interventions and actions for a client receiving oxytocin augmentation?

5. Two hours after infusion, Mrs. M. is receiving eight mcg/min of oxytocin. The FHR is 150 bpm. Her contractions are every two to three minutes and lasting 60–90 seconds. All maternal vital signs are within normal limits. What is your analysis of this data?

6. After three hours, there appear to be signs of fetal bradycardia coupled with an elevation in maternal blood pressure. What priority nursing interventions should be initiated at this time?

MULTIPLE CHOICE

1. The term that indicates that the largest diameter of the presenting part has passed through the inlet into the true pelvis is known as _____.

   A. engagement   C. effacement
   B. station   D. presentation

2. The most common type of female pelvis is the _____ type.

   A. android   C. gynecoid
   B. anthropoid   D. platypelloid

3. The phase of labor that begins with the onset of regular, mild contractions is known as the _____.

   A. latent phase
   B. active phase
   C. transition phase
   D. pushing phase

4. The average length of the transition phase for a multigravida is _____.

   A. 30 minutes
   B. one hour
   C. two hours
   D. three hours

5. A type of synthetic prostaglandin, which is normally used for the treatment of peptic ulcer disease but may also be utilized for the induction of labor, is called _____.

   A. pitocin
   B. prepidil
   C. cervidil
   D. cytotec

MULTIPLE RESPONSE

1. Lightening is the movement of the presenting body part into the true pelvis. Which of the following are descriptions of what a pregnant client might report feeling after lightening occurs? Select all that apply.

   A. painless, irregular contractions felt in the front of the abdomen
   B. a feeling of being able to breathe more easily
   C. blood-tinged secretions from the vagina
   D. edema of the lower extremities
   E. increased urinary frequency

2. Which of the following is considered a cardinal movement of labor? Select all that apply.

   A. descent
   B. flexion
   C. dilation
   D. crowning
   E. expulsion

3. Which of the following are contraindications for labor induction? Select all that apply.

   A. placenta previa
   B. postterm gestation
   C. intrauterine growth restriction
   D. transverse fetal lie
   E. active herpes infection

CHAPTER 15

Nursing Care of the Intrapartal Family

KEY TERMS

Please define the following terms:

Acrocyanosis

Amnioinfusion

Apgar score

Bloody show

Chorioamnionitis

Contraction

Crowning

Dilation

Duration

Effacement

Emergency childbirth

Episiotomy

Fern test

Gravidity

Hyperventilation

Intensity

Intrauterine pressure catheter (IUPC)

Inversion of the uterus

Labor

Laceration

Meconium

Montevideo unit

Multipara

Nitrazine test

Nuchal cord

Oligohydramnios

Parity

Parturient

Placenta previa

Polyhydramnios

Precipitous delivery

Premature rupture of membranes (PROM)

Presenting part

Preterm birth

Preterm premature rupture of membranes (PPROM)

Reactive non-stress test

Resting tone

Second stage labor

Station

Striae gravidarum

Third stage labor

True labor

Uterine atony

Vertex

ACTIVITIES

1. Review the questions the nurse should ask the pregnant client. Explain why the question is important and what information is sought.

   What is your reason for coming to the hospital?

   When is your baby due?

   How many babies have you had?

   When did your labor begin?

   Has the bag of water (membranes) broken? What time? What color was the fluid? Have you noticed any bleeding?

   How has your pregnancy been? Have you been hospitalized during this pregnancy? Is there anything about you or your pregnancy that I should know?

   Are you allergic to any food or medications that you know of? Are you allergic to latex? Have you ever had a bad reaction to medications, latex, or blood?

2. What is the focus of initial admission observations?

3. What is the importance of the nurse asking the color of the fluid if the "bag of water" (i.e., membranes) broke?

4. Why is it important for the informed consent form to be signed prior to the client being administered medications?

5. List three major categories/conditions that put the client at increased risk during pregnancy.

6. Differentiate gravidity and parity.

7. Discuss pregnancy risk factors identified from the mother's history.

8. Compare the five-digit method and the two-digit method in documenting gravidity and parity.

9. Name problems of particular importance a nurse should be informed of.

10. List chronic illnesses noted in the text that would put the client and fetus at great risk.

11. State the health risks associated with smoking during pregnancy.

12. Describe the results of anxiety and high levels of stress during pregnancy.

13. Discuss the nurse's responsibility in domestic violence screening.

14. Discuss the use of the electronic fetal monitor and auscultation for fetal heart tones.

15. State the classification (range) of FHRs:
    Normal

    Tachycardia

    Bradycardia

16. Compare the tocotransducer and the IUPC.

17. State the risk of rupture of the membranes and a delay of more than 24 hours to birth.

18. Compare the nitrazine and fern tests.

19. Explain station of the presenting part of the fetus in relation to the maternal pelvis.

20. Define hypertension in the laboring mother.

21. Define the presence of swelling, redness, and a positive Homan's sign when examining the lower extremities.

22. Describe clonus.

23. Discuss the presence of epigastric or right upper quadrant pain.

24. Describe the stages and phases of labor.

25. Explain the importance of taking vital signs of the mother in labor.

26. Compare long-term variability, short-term (or beat-to-beat) variability, periodic, and non-periodic heart rate changes.

27. Define acceleration and deceleration of FHRs. Explain how decelerations are classified.

28. Discuss the interventions for non-reassuring FHR patterns.

29. Discuss hydration of the client in labor:
   Oral fluid

   Intravenous fluids

30. Define amniotomy, amniohook, and the nursing responsibilities before and after the procedure.

31. Discuss the importance of documentation and communication by the labor and delivery nurse.

32. Discuss anxiety levels and coping mechanisms of the client and her support system.

33. Describe how the demeanor of the nurse may affect the client throughout her birthing experience.

34. Explain pain relief during the labor process.

35. Define the advantages and disadvantages of a doula.

36. Discuss psychologic considerations and their effects on the mother in labor.

37. Explain the labor curve.

38. Define primary power and secondary power in the second stage of labor.

39. Describe the pushing technique.

40. Describe meconium aspiration and the procedures used by the delivery room personnel to correct this.

41. Complete the Apgar scoring system:

	Score		
Sign	0	1	2

42. Describe the newborn evaluation at delivery.

43. Describe the identification process for the newborn and the mother.

44. Discuss the possible results of attempts to prematurely deliver the placenta, and of inversion of the uterus.

45. Define the fourth stage of labor.

46. Compare positive and negative maternal bonding.

47. Define when oxytocin is given and its purpose.

48. Explain the standardized method for estimating lochia after delivery:

    Scant

    Light

    Moderate

    Heavy

49. Discuss the factors associated with postpartum uterine atony.

50. Explain the importance of instructing the new mother in palpating her uterus.

51. Discuss nursing interventions during a precipitous delivery.

SELF-ASSESSMENT QUIZ

1. True or False

   T   F   It is the nurse's responsibility to give the client information and rationale for interventions that may be performed, including risks and alternatives.

   T   F   The nurse obtains and witnesses the client's signature on the consent form.

   T   F   Complete effacement and delivery of the baby signal the end of the first stage of labor.

   T   F   Premature pushing will cause the cervix to swell and impede labor.

   T   F   Full dilation of the cervix is a function of descent.

   T   F   The most commonly used position in the United States for pushing in the second stage of labor is the Sims' position.

2. The informed consent form should include emergency procedures that may prove necessary. List them.

3. What food types should a client who has phenylketonuria (PKU) be advised not to consume?

4. State the importance of acquiring information of any uterine surgeries.

5. List chronic illnesses that would place additional burden on the pregnant mother.

6. State the importance of acquiring demographic and psychosocial information.

7. Differentiate between frequency and duration of contractions.

8. Compare polyhydramnios and oligohydramnios. State the amount of milliliters the uterus contains at the end of pregnancy.

9. Compare effacement and dilation.

10. Describe the steps taken to check for Homan's sign.

11. State the two cardinal signs of pre-eclampsia.

12. Describe periorbital edema.

13. Discuss findings of a urinalysis regarding albuminuria, glucose, and ketones.

14. Describe the blood tests given during labor.

15. Describe "laboring down."

16. Differentiate between the passive and active phases of the second stage of labor.

17. Define crowning.

18. Identify the procedure used to shorten the second stage of labor.

19. Define nuchal cord.

20. Define shoulder dystocia.

21. Describe the two "breathing patterns" of the fetus in utero by which it moves amniotic fluid into and out of the lungs.

22. Describe acrocyanosis and the length of **time** it may persist.

23. State the time elements the Apgar score uses to evaluate the neonate.

24. Explain the cause of a displaced fundus.

25. Define a boggy uterus.

26. Identify the position of the fundus at the fourth stage of labor.

27. Define lochia.

28. Identify causes of continuous bleeding in a firm, contracted uterus.

CRITICAL THINKING

1. Some labor room nurses have a hard time accepting that a client chooses not to have any pharmacological pain relief in labor and delivery. What do you think the reason for this attitude might be?

2. A childbirth coach can sometimes be made to feel "in the way." How can you make the coach feel more welcome and comfortable?

3. Draw a fetus inside a uterus. Draw the fetus in a longitudinal lie, cephalic lie, and extended attitude.

MULTIPLE CHOICE

1. According to the GTPAL method of determining gravidity and parity for the pregnant client, a woman who presents as a G5P3013 has had how many preterm babies?

   A. five
   B. three

   C. one
   D. zero

2. When the presenting part is seen at the woman's perineum, it is said to be at what station?

   A. +3
   B. +1

   C. 0
   D. -1

3. Which of the following should be considered if the client presents with bright red vaginal bleeding?

   A. performing a sterile vaginal examination
   B. notifying the primary care provider
   C. performing Leopold's maneuver
   D. checking the client's temperature

4. When assessing pre-tibial edema, a 3+ assessment of the client includes which of the following?

   A. a sense of fullness
   B. blanching of the skin and depression
   C. small suggestion of fullness
   D. indentation remains and gradually recedes

5. Which of the following is a nursing intervention that should be implemented for non-reassuring fetal heart tones?

   A. Place the patient in the Trendelenburg position.
   B. Start oxygen therapy by nasal cannula at one liter per minute.
   C. Increase the rate of the main IV line.
   D. Anticipate administration of oxytocin.

MULTIPLE CHOICE

1. Which of the following are indications of true labor? Select all that apply.

   A. Lying down lengthens the interval of contractions.
   B. The cervix dilates and becomes effaced.
   C. Bloody show is absent.
   D. Contraction intervals shorten.
   E. Contractions increase with walking.

2. Which of the following are priority assessments for the woman who is admitted in an advanced stage of labor? Select all that apply.

   A. Is there a language barrier?
   B. Does the woman avoid eye contact?
   C. Does the woman have insurance?
   D. Is the woman able to ask for what she needs?
   E. Is there a doula present?

3. Besides the cardinal indicators of pre-eclampsia, hypertension, and proteinuria, which of the following may also be potential signs of the illness? Select all that apply.

   A. visual disturbances
   B. sluggish deep tendon reflexes
   C. epigastric pain
   D. headache
   E. positive Homan's sign

CHAPTER 16

High-Risk Births and Obstetric Emergencies

KEY TERMS

Please define the following terms:

Abruptio placentae

Amniotic fluid embolism

Amniotomy

Anencephaly

Breech presentation

Brow presentation

Cephalopelvic disproportion (CPD)

Contracted maternal pelvis

Dysfunctional labor pattern

External cephalic version

Face presentation

Fetal distress

Hydrocephalus

Hypertonic labor

Hypotonic labor

Intrauterine pressure catheter (IUPC)

Kleihauer-Betke test

Labor augmentation

Malposition

Malpresentation

Multiple gestation

Oligohydramnios

Placenta percreta

Placenta previa

Polyhydramnios

Precipitate labor

Shoulder dystocia

Shoulder presentation

Transverse lie

Turtle sign

Umbilical cord compression

Umbilical cord prolapse

Uterine rupture

Vasa previa

Velamentous insertion of the cord

ACTIVITIES

1. Identify the following fetal monitoring terms and parameters:

Baseline Data

Data	Defining Characteristics
Rate	
Normal	

Tachycardia

Bradycardia

Variability

Short-term

Long-term

Rhythm

Regular

Irregular

Periodic Changes

Data	Defining Characteristics
Accelerations	
Decelerations	
Variable	
Early	
Late	
Prolonged	

---

2. How do anxiety and pain affect the labor process?

3. Discuss oxytocin augmentation of labor.

4. Differentiate between hypertonic and hypotonic labor by completing the following table:

	Hypertonic	Hypotonic
Contributing factors		
Consequences		
Assessment findings		
Treatment		
Nursing diagnoses		
Outcomes		

5. Discuss precipitate labor and delivery.

6. Differentiate between malpresentation and malposition.

7. Propose a nursing plan of care for a client with malpresentation.

8. List contributing factors for cephalopelvic disproportion.

9. What maternal factors increase the risk of macrosomia?

10. Describe the turtle sign.

11. Explain the McRoberts maneuver.

12. Differentiate between the Woods corkscrew maneuver and the Rubin maneuver. When would these maneuvers be indicated?

13. What are common complications of multiple gestation pregnancies?

14. Discuss the nurse's role in caring for a client with multiple gestational pregnancy.

15. Define fetal distress. What are the possible complications of fetal distress?

16. Differentiate between a reactive and a non-reactive non-stress test.

17. List interventions to increase fetal oxygenation.

18. Paraphrase the procedure for amnioinfusion.

19. Your pregnant client has had blunt trauma to the abdomen. What signs and symptoms would help you to recognize uterine rupture? What are the maternal complications? What are the fetal complications?

20. Differentiate the following abnormalities:

	Placenta Previa	Abruptio Placentae	Umbilical Cord Compression	Umbilical Cord Prolapse
Definition				
Risk factors				
Assessment findings				
Maternal complications				
Fetal complications				
Treatment				
Nursing diagnoses				
Nursing interventions				
Outcomes				

21. Differentiate between polyhydramnios and oligohydramnios. What are the complications of each? Describe the treatment.

SELF-ASSESSMENT QUIZ

1. The drug used for labor augmentation is _____.

2. True or False

    T   F   The leading cause of primary cesarean sections is dysfunctional labor.

    T   F   A fetal heart rate over 160 bpm is considered tachycardia.

    T   F   Amniotomy may be used to augment labor.

    T   F   Hypotonic labor refers to uterine contractions that are inadequate in frequency, intensity, and duration.

3. Two major risks in multiple gestation pregnancies are _____ and _____.

CRITICAL THINKING

Mrs. L., a 39-year-old primigravida, was admitted to the nursing unit in active labor 26 hours ago. She had been diagnosed with gestational diabetes at 26 weeks' gestation and has mild chronic hypertension. Based on ultrasound, her baby weighs approximately four kg. Currently, she is ten centimeters dilated and has been pushing for almost two hours. You observe that the fetal head retracts after each push. There is pronounced caput, and the fetal head remains at zero station.

1. What obstetrical emergency is this client at risk for?

2. What are this particular client's risk factors for an obstetrical emergency? The fetal head is delivered 30 minutes later and shoulder dystocia is diagnosed.

3. List all critical nursing responsibilities at this time.

4. Describe the McRoberts maneuver and suprapubic pressure. Seven minutes later the infant is delivered and his Apgar scores are three and seven.

5. What is your priority nursing diagnosis for the infant at this time?

6. Discuss risks to the mother that are associated with a difficult shoulder dystocia.

MULTIPLE CHOICE

1. Women who experience intense, precipitous labor are at increased risk for
_____.

   A. infection
   B. amniotic fluid embolism
   C. low blood pressure
   D. umbilical cord prolapse

2. A condition that causes increased circulating cerebrospinal fluid resulting in a larger fetal head is known as _____.

   A. anencephaly
   B. cephalohematoma
   C. hydrocephalus
   D. occipitocephalic dystocia

3. Which of the following is a form of medical management for brow presentation?

   A. oxytocin augmentation
   B. midpelvic manipulation
   C. emergency cesarean section
   D. epidural anesthesia

4. Which of the following conditions may contribute to uterine rupture?

   A. advanced maternal age
   B. blunt trauma
   C. primiparity
   D. hypertension

5. A condition that occurs when the umbilical cord crosses the cervical os is known as _____.

   A. placenta previa
   B. velamentous insertion of the cord
   C. umbilical cord prolapse
   D. vasa previa

MULTIPLE RESPONSE

1. Which of the following are factors that contribute to hypertonic labor? Select all that apply.

   A. prematurity
   B. primiparous labor
   C. fetal presentation other than cephalic
   D. increased fetal size
   E. premature rupture of membranes

2. Which of the following circumstances are common indications for cesarean delivery? Select all that apply.

   A. footling presentation
   B. occipitoanterior position
   C. macrosomia
   D. request for sterilization
   E. precipitate labor

3. Which of the following are risk factors for the fetus with macrosomia? Select all that apply.

   A. Klumpke's palsy
   B. infection
   C. stillbirth
   D. shoulder dystocia
   E. clavicle fracture

CHAPTER 17

Pain Management in Labor and Delivery: Analgesia and Anesthesia

KEY TERMS

Please define the following terms:

Analgesia

Anesthesia

Dermatome

Doula

Epidural anesthesia

General anesthesia

Local anesthetic

Local infiltration anesthesia

Parenteral

Pudendal block

Regional anesthesia

Spinal anesthesia

ACTIVITIES

1. Recall the three anesthesia techniques.

2. Discuss theories of pain and pain management.

3. Who are the members of the anesthesia care team?

4. What mechanisms cause pain in various stages of labor?

5. Recall the pros and cons of parenteral analgesia.

6. What actions should be taken for a neonate with opioid-induced depression?

7. What is the purpose of midazolam (Versed) during labor and delivery?

8. Formulate your personal definition of pain. Compare your definition to that of your lab partner.

9. Discuss nursing responsibilities for a client undergoing intrathecal or epidural anesthesia.

10. Explain how to position a client for insertion of an epidural catheter.

11. List advantages and disadvantages of epidural analgesia.

Advantages	Disadvantages

12. List absolute and relative contraindications to regional analgesia and anesthesia.

Absolute Contraindication	Relative Contraindication

13. List side effects and complications of epidural analgesia.

14. List risk factors associated with postdural headache.

15. Differentiate between postdural headache and headache associated with postpartum recovery.

16. Discuss independent and collaborative treatment of postdural headache.

17. List advantages and disadvantages of general anesthesia.

Advantages	Disadvantages

18. Discuss the postoperative care of the client who has had anesthesia.

Local

Regional

General

SELF-ASSESSMENT QUIZ

1. At what level does the spinal cord end?

2. Which type of anesthesia during labor has the least complications?

3. Which type of anesthesia is suitable for all types of delivery?

4. When is it safe for the nurse to relieve cricoid pressure when assisting with intubation?

CRITICAL THINKING

Mrs. M. is a 28-year-old G2P1 who presents to the labor unit for delivery. Her initial assessment shows her amniotic membranes are intact and her cervix is dilated to three centimeters. Mrs. M. requests that she initially be allowed to labor without the use of pharmacologic pain methods.

1. What are the physiologic changes occurring during this time that might be causing pain for Mrs. M.?

2. What non-pharmacologic methods of pain control can the nurse provide for Mrs. M.?

   After two hours of labor, Mrs. M. is rating her pain at a "seven" on a pain scale of zero to ten. Her amniotic membranes have ruptured after she spent the last two hours walking, and her cervix is dilated to five centimeters. She requests medication for pain control at this time.

3. What are Mrs. M.'s options at this point for pharmacologic pain control?

Mrs. M. reaches the second stage of labor and begins to push. Because the baby's head is stretching the perineum, the physician performs an episiotomy to allow room for delivery without causing a laceration.

4. What pain control options are necessary for an episiotomy?

5. Following delivery, what nursing interventions are necessary to care for Mrs. M. as she recovers?

MULTIPLE CHOICE

1. Which of the following physicians developed a method of delivery known as "husband-coached childbirth?"

   A. Marjorie Kimmel
   B. Ferdinand Lamaze
   C. Robert A. Bradley
   D. Grantley Dick-Read

2. Which of the following is true regarding hydrotherapy?

   A. With hydrotherapy, the nurse must perform a vaginal examination every 30 minutes while the client is in the water.
   B. Bathing is associated with increased speed of cervical dilation.
   C. Hydrotherapy cannot be used for multiparous women.
   D. When using hydrotherapy, the woman must get out of the water after she has reached five centimeters of cervical dilation.

3. A subarachnoid block is considered to be which form of pain control?

    A. analgesia   C. general anesthesia

    B. local anesthesia   D. regional anesthesia

4. Which of the following is a type of opioid analgesic used for pain control during labor and delivery?

    A. Phenergen   C. Vistaril

    B. Demerol   D. Versed

5. Which of the following is an absolute contraindication for regional anesthesia?

    A. hemorrhage   C. spinal deformity

    B. sepsis   D. heparinization

MULTIPLE RESPONSE

1. Which of the following are types of factors that may influence pain for a laboring client? Select all that apply.

    A. age

    B. fear

    C. marital status

    D. cultural beliefs

    E. anxiety

2. Which of the following are true about sterile water injections? Select all that apply.

    A. Sterile water injections are designed to relieve severe back pain.

    B. Upper sterile water injections are placed over the posterior superior iliac spines.

    C. With sterile water injections, each area is injected intradermally with ten milliliters of sterile water.

    D. Staff nurses typically provide sterile water injections as a form of pain relief.

    E. Women can expect 60 to 90 minutes of back pain relief with sterile water injections.

3. During the first stage of labor, which of the following are reasons the woman may experience pain? Select all that apply.

    A. cervical dilation

    B. uterine contractions

    C. exhaustion

    D. distention of the vagina

    E. pressure on the sacrum

UNIT 6
Postpartum Nursing Care

CHAPTER 18

Nursing Care of the Low-Risk Postpartum Family

KEY TERMS

Please define the following terms:

Afterpains

Atony

Attachment

Boggy

Diastasis recti

Endometritis

Engorgement

Episiotomy

Fundus

Involution

Letting-go phase

Lochia

Maternal-infant bonding

Puerperium

Residual urine

Role attainment

Role transition

Sleep-wake cycle

Striae gravidarum

Subinvolution

Taking-hold phase

Taking-in phase

ACTIVITIES

1. Describe the client's blood pressure in the immediate and early postpartum period. What signs should the nurse be alerted to for hemorrhage?

2. Describe the client's pulse, respiratory rate, and temperature in the postpartum period.

3. Explain the cause of shivers or tremors immediately post-delivery.

4. Describe assessment of postpartum bleeding.

5. Explain and summarize fundal massage.

6. Describe the criteria for straight catheterization of a postpartum client.

7. Summarize the physical postpartum assessment BUBBLE-HE.

   Breasts

   Uterine fundus

   Bladder

   Bowel

   Lochia
     Rubra

     Serosa

     Alba

Episiotomy

Homan's sign

Emotional status

8. Propose a plan to assist the postpartum client who has had an episiotomy, hemorrhoids, and is constipated.

9. Identify the three types of lochia and their duration.

10. Explain the warning sign of a boggy or soft uterus. What could this indicate?

11. Describe the care of the episiotomy and vulva.

12. List and describe perineal lacerations.

13. Identify the nursing care for a client with an episiotomy.

14. Describe assessing for Homan's sign.

15. Summarize client education to the postpartum client. Include general discharge instructions, warning signs of later hemorrhage, and signs of illness.

16. Develop a plan for discharging postpartum clients. Incorporate referrals, visiting nurses, and infant care issues, along with any other important information for the client.

17. Describe nursing interventions to promote maternal-infant bonding.

18. Complete the following table on maternal-infant adjustment according to Rubin:

Phase	Title	Maternal Characteristics	Examples	Nursing Responsibilities

19. List nursing interventions to promote attachment behaviors.

20. Formulate nursing interventions to assist parental role adjustment.

21. Describe infant behaviors that influence attachment.

22. Using a lab partner, practice communicating with a child experiencing sibling adjustment. Offer interventions to promote adjustment.

23. What factors can affect the role of the grandparents? How can grandparents be included in the family adjustment?

24. Propose nursing diagnoses that may be appropriate for postpartum family adjustment.

SELF-ASSESSMENT QUIZ

1. Match the following terms with their definitions.

   _____ Puerperium   A. Uterus reducing in size

   _____ Engorgement   B. Not firm or palpable

   _____ Residual urine   C. Infection of uterine lining

   _____ Subinvolution   D. Loss of muscle tone

   _____ Striae   E. Postpartum period

   _____ Lochia   F. Surgical incision made to enlarge the vaginal opening

   _____ Involution   G. Urine remaining in the bladder after elimination

   _____ Endometritis   H. Failure of the uterus to return to a non-pregnant state

   _____ Atony   I. Enlargement and filling of the breasts with milk

   _____ Boggy uterus   J. Stretch marks

   _____ Episiotomy   K. Uterine discharge of blood and tissue after childbirth

2. Describe the time frame of the postpartum period.

3. State the difference in healing time between primiparas and multiparas.

4. Describe the average weight loss for a client post-delivery.

5. RhoGam immunizations are given postpartum to which eligible mother at what time interval?

6. List four attachment behaviors that initiate attachment interactions between an infant and the mother.

7. Indicate whether the following maternal characteristics are (1) initial phase: taking-in phase; (2) second phase: taking-hold phase; or (3) third phase: letting-go phase, according to Rubin's theory.

_____ Mother resumes control over her life

_____ Maternal role attainment

_____ Mother begins to gain self-confidence

_____ Relationship adjustment

_____ Preoccupation with self

_____ Compares child with "fantasy child"

_____ Concerned about self-care

_____ Interested in caring for her newborn

8. True or False

T   F   Self-esteem is a major predictor for maternal role competence for both primiparas and multiparas.

T   F   Paternal involvement is a significant factor in fostering a positive interaction between adolescent mothers and their children.

9. List five ways the nurse can promote maternal attachment behaviors.

CRITICAL THINKING

Marta is 12 hours postpartum following a 16-hour labor and delivery. She had a normal vaginal birth with a first-degree laceration.

Objective Data

Fundus firm, midline @ umbilicus with moderate bright red lochia

Vital signs: temp. 38C, pulse 85, resp. 22, BP 100/60

Laboratory results: Rh status positive, Coombs negative, Rubella titer negative, Hematocrit 33%

You find Marta happily talking on the phone when you enter her room. She is recounting the details of her labor and does not appear interested in her baby. She asks you to butter her toast, even though she appears perfectly capable of doing this task.

1. What is your best analysis of this behavior?

2. How would you respond to Marta?

3. You are performing a routine postpartum assessment on Marta. What should be included?

4. Should Marta receive any vaccinations at this point?

5. One hour post-delivery, Marta's fundus is boggy and deviated to the left of the umbilicus. What are your priority interventions and assessments?

6. You return in 30 minutes to reassess Marta. Although her fundus is now midline, it is still boggy and her perineal pad is saturated. What are the possibilities?

7. What are the most common reasons for postpartum hemorrhage?

MULTIPLE CHOICE

1. What period of time is considered to be the early postpartum period?

   A. the first hour after delivery
   B. the first 24 hours after delivery
   C. the second day after birth to the end of the first week
   D. the first six weeks

2. Which of the following is a risk factor for a urinary tract infection in the postpartum period?

   A. frequent vaginal exams during labor
   B. intrapartum fever
   C. prolonged rupture of membranes
   D. anxiety

3. Twelve hours after delivery, the nurse palpates a client's fundus and finds that it is midline and located approximately one centimeter below the level of the umbilicus. What sign does this indicate?

   A. retained urine in the bladder
   B. uterine atony
   C. retained placental fragments
   D. a normal finding

4. Which of the following are indications for performing a straight catheterization on a postpartum client?

   A. blood pressure 100/60
   B. midline fundus approximately one centimeter below the umbilicus

   C. palpable bladder
   D. moderate lochia rubra

5. How can the nurse encourage the client who is constipated and hesitant to defecate because of a fourth degree laceration?

   A. Administer Tylenol with codeine for pain relief.
   B. Allow the client to use a warm sitz bath.
   C. Administer an enema to relieve constipation.
   D. Encourage the client to cut back on drinking liquids.

MULTIPLE RESPONSE

1. Which of the following are benefits of mother-baby nursing for the family and newborn? Select all that apply.

   A. fostering breastfeeding
   B. promoting the grandmother's role and attachment
   C. promoting the mother's self-care capabilities
   D. promoting duplication of services
   E. decreasing the incidence of cross-infection

2. Which of the following are common signs of postpartum hemorrhage? Select all that apply.

   A. low blood pressure
   B. perineal laceration
   C. uterine atony
   D. retained placenta
   E. temperature of 100.2° F

3. Which of the following are considered methods of suppression of lactation for the woman who chooses to bottle-feed her infant? Select all that apply.

   A. palpating the breasts every four hours
   B. binding the breasts with a support bra
   C. taking a hot shower
   D. expressing breast milk when breasts feel full
   E. applying ice packs to the breasts

CHAPTER 19

Complications of Postpartum and Neonatal Loss

KEY TERMS

Please define the following terms:

Anticipatory grieving

Atony

Grief

Grief work

Mastitis

Pathologic grief

Puerperal sepsis

Relinquishment

Reproductive loss

Sudden infant death syndrome (SIDS)

ACTIVITIES

1. List the causes for early hemorrhage.

2. Discuss the risk factors for uterine atony.

3. Describe the types of postpartum hemorrhage and their severity.

4. Discuss and categorize four types of puerperal hematomas.

5. Describe the risk factors for postpartum infections.

6. Define mastitis, its causes, and client teaching.

7. Describe the emotions experienced by the pregnant mother when loss occurs at any of the stages of pregnancy.

8. Identify and discuss the three components of grief work.

9. Interview administrative members of a support group on grief to see how different couples cope with their individual situation.

10. Discuss the nurse's role in relinquishment.

SELF-ASSESSMENT QUIZ

1. List the medications used to control postpartum hemorrhage or heavy bleeding.

2. Explain the dangers if the third stage of labor is mismanaged.

3. State the most common reason for postpartum hemorrhage.

4. Identify the four stages of grief identified by Davidson.

5. Describe the nurse's role when the mother is to relinquish her child.

6. List the types of grief parents may experience.

CRITICAL THINKING

1. Liza is a 29-year-old woman who delivered her first baby ten days ago. Her son was born at 32 weeks' gestation, and although he is small, he is stable and doing well in the neonatal intensive care unit (NICU). She visits her baby as often as the hospital allows. Her husband appears very supportive, but he works long hours and is unable to accompany Liza most of the time. While caring for the baby, you observe that Liza frequently appears tearful and upset. On one visit, Liza's husband takes you aside and tells you he is very concerned about his wife's welfare. He claims she has not been eating or sleeping the last three to four days. The nurses in the NICU decide to have a team meeting to discuss Liza and develop a plan of action.

   a. What are your thoughts? What are some of the likely reasons for Liza's behaviors?

   b. What disciplines should members of this team be from?

   c. What additional assessments would be appropriate at this time?

d. Compare and contrast postpartum blues, postpartum depression (PPD), and postpartum psychosis (PPP).

e. Discuss the medical management of PPP.

2. When caring for a client after delivery, the nurse notes an excessive rubra flow with large clots.

a. Identify the nurse's priority action in response to the assessment finding.

b. In order of priority, what are the most common risk factors for postpartum hemorrhage?

MULTIPLE CHOICE

1. Hypothermia that occurs during hemorrhagic shock is a result of _____.

   A. systemic vasoconstriction
   B. decreased metabolism
   C. extracellular fluid
   D. reduced renal perfusion

2. Which of the following is a symptom that occurs during stage two of postpartum hemorrhage?

   A. tachycardia
   B. agitation
   C. hemodynamic instability
   D. confusion

3. Which of the following is a clinical finding associated with endometritis?

   A. warmth and swelling
   B. anemia
   C. gastrointestinal distress
   D. positive Homan's sign

4. Which of the following is a risk factor for postpartum blues?

   A. history of previous postpartum psychosis
   B. history of abuse
   C. adverse reactions to oral contraceptives
   D. primiparity

5. Which of the following are characteristics of the searching and yearning stage of grief?

   A. extreme sensitivity to stimuli
   B. anorexia
   C. restlessness and impatience
   D. sense of release

MULTIPLE RESPONSE

1. Which of the following are risk factors for uterine atony? Select all that apply.

   A. bicornate uterus
   B. small blood clots
   C. presence of fibroids
   D. prematurity
   E. polyhydramnios

2. Which of the following are nursing interventions for the client with a urinary tract infection (UTI)? Select all that apply.

   A. Encourage the client to avoid sleeping on her stomach.
   B. Provide comfort measures such as sitz baths.
   C. Provide analgesia as necessary.
   D. Encourage the client to avoid carbonated drinks.
   E. Encourage increased fluid intake.

3. Which of the following is a true statement about mastitis? Select all that apply.

   A. The nurse should apply ice packs to the affected breast.
   B. The nurse should encourage the client to change to bottle feeding.
   C. The client requires ample fluids and plenty of rest.
   D. Mastitis can occur as early as one to three days postpartum.
   E. The client may experience flu-like symptoms such as nausea, vomiting, and chills.

CHAPTER 20

Lactation and Newborn Nutrition

KEY TERMS

Please define the following terms:

Alveoli

Antioxidant

Areola

Bioavailability

Colostrum

Engorgement

Foremilk

Galactopoiesis

Hindmilk

Lactation consultant

Lactogenesis

La Leche League

Latching-on

Let-down reflex

Macronutrients

Mammogenesis

Mastitis

Mature milk

Micronutrients

Oxytocin

Prolactin

Reducing agent

Renal solute load

Rooting reflex

Transitional milk

Weaning

ACTIVITIES

1. Explain the hormonal control of lactation in the following categories:

   Mammogenesis

   Lactogenesis

2. Discuss the role of hormones in lactation.

3. Define the let-down reflex.

4. Describe the many factors that can interfere with the lactation process.

5. Summarize how the interference of the following factors may influence breastfeeding:

   Anxiety

   Medical problems

   Nutritional and fluid intake

6. Describe the importance of the nurse's role in assisting new mothers in all aspects of breastfeeding (without the mother having feelings of inadequacy).

7. Define rooting reflex and latching-on and their importance in lactation.

8. Explain the long-term benefits of breastfeeding.

9. Explain the immunologic benefits of breastfeeding.

10. Define the following barriers to lactation:
    Biologic barriers

    Psychological barriers

    Social barriers

11. Differentiate among the following biologic barriers:
    Maternal barriers

    Nipple inversion

    Nipple sensitivity

    Hormonal barriers

    Decreased lactogenesis

12. Differentiate among the following infant barriers:
    Prematurity

    Illness and disability

    Hypoglycemia

    Jaundice

13. Differentiate between the following psychological barriers:
    Modesty

Lack of confidence

14. Differentiate between the following social barriers:
Lack of social support

Misperceptions and misconceptions

15. Define the following additional barriers to breastfeeding:
Hospital policies

Return to work

16. Interview a lactating mother and inquire about her feelings and attitude about breastfeeding.

17. Discuss contraindications in breastfeeding:
Maternal disease

Infant disease

Drugs and medications

18. Explain the following maternal problems encountered with breastfeeding:
Cracked or sore nipples

Inverted nipples

Breast engorgement

Mastitis

19. Differentiate among alternative therapies for breastfeeding problems.

20. Summarize how a lactating mother, upon returning to work, pumps, stores, and supplements her breast milk.

21. Discuss the resources available for breastfeeding mothers.

22. Explain how education and cultural negotiations help the lactating mother overcome barriers.

23. Discuss the importance of the first feeding.

24. Summarize the nursing process in assisting the lactating mother to achieve success in breastfeeding.

25. Compare the contents of human milk and commercial formulas by completing the table:

	Amount	Characteristics	Implications	Requirements
Breast milk				
Kcal				
Protein				
Fat				
Carbohydrate				
Na				
K				

Ca

Fe

Formula (standard cow's milk)

Kcal

Protein

Fat

Carbohydrate

Na

K

Ca

Fe

_____

26. Differentiate between macronutrients and micronutrients.

27. What substances are considered trace elements?

28. At what age does an infant require iron from a dietary source?

29. Complete the following table on water-soluble vitamins:

Vitamin	Requirements 0–6 Months	Requirements 6–12 Months	Actions
Vitamin C			
Thiamin			
Riboflavin			
Niacin			
Vitamin B$_6$			
Folate			
Vitamin B$_{12}$			

30. Complete the following table on fat-soluble vitamins:

Vitamin	Requirements 0–6 Months	Requirements 6–12 Months	Actions
Vitamin A			
Vitamin D			
Vitamin E			
Vitamin K			

31. Compare the terms lactation and breastfeeding.

32. What factors influence a mother's decision to breastfeed?

33. Categorize commercially available infant formulas. Describe the criteria used to classify them.

34. List the symptoms of food allergies.

35. Describe how preterm infant formulas differ from term infant formulas.

36. Discuss indications and methods for sterilizing infant formulas and equipment.

SELF-ASSESSMENT QUIZ

1. Breastfeeding mothers will need approximately _____ extra calories daily.

2. State the importance of colostrum for the new infant.

3. True or False

    T   F   Colostrum is regarded as "old" milk and is not utilized in some societies.

    T   F   Breastfeeding acts as a natural birth control method.

    T   F   The decision to stop breastfeeding is called relactation.

    T   F   Hindmilk is thin and watery.

    T   F   The most effective time to prepare for breastfeeding is early in the prenatal period.

4. List the cellular components of human milk.

5. Define the following categories of breast milk:

    Transitional milk

    Foremilk

    Hindmilk

    Mature milk

6. List three benefits of breastfeeding.

7. Describe six behaviors an infant might display when hungry.

8. Indicate whether the following vitamins are (1) water soluble or (2) fat soluble:

_____ Vitamin C

_____ Vitamin D

_____ Vitamin K

_____ Vitamin B$_{12}$

_____ Thiamin

_____ Niacin

_____ Vitamin E

_____ Vitamin A

9. At what age should solid food be introduced to an infant?

CRITICAL THINKING

Barbara is a brand new mother who delivered a healthy term baby three hours ago following a 12-hour labor and an uncomplicated vaginal birth. When asked about feeding her baby, Barbara tells you she is not convinced that breastfeeding is really worth all the effort and fuss. She is worried about "ruining her figure" and not getting a break from the baby.

1. What additional assessments would be appropriate at this time?

2. Respond to Barbara's concerns regarding "ruining her figure" and not getting a break from the baby.

3. Describe the benefits of breastfeeding to the mother.

4. List and describe the assessments you would perform on the baby to determine readiness.

5. Describe to the mother the benefits of breastfeeding the baby.

6. Explain any anticipated drawbacks or barriers to breastfeeding.

7. Develop goals and interventions that will lead the mother to successful breastfeeding outcomes. Include short-term and long-term goals.

MULTIPLE CHOICE

1. The fats in human milk provide approximately _____ percent of calories in the milk.

   A. 15 percent
   B. 25 percent
   C. 50 percent
   D. 90 percent

2. A substance that slows down the negative effects of hydrocarbons, oils, and fats, thus helping to check deterioration is called a(n) _____.

   A. reducing agent
   B. antioxidant
   C. water-soluble vitamin
   D. fat-soluble vitamin

3. A type of vitamin that is unique among nutrients because the body can synthesize it with exposure to sunlight is called _____.

   A. Vitamin A
   B. Vitamin B_6
   C. Vitamin C
   D. Vitamin D

4. The maintenance of established milk secretion during breastfeeding is known as _____.

   A. lactogenesis I
   B. lactogenesis II
   C. mammogenesis
   D. galactopoiesis

5. The best type of breast-feeding position that offers visibility and is excellent for a baby with low tone would be the _____.

    A. cradle hold   C. football hold
    B. cross cradle hold   D. side-lying hold

MULTIPLE RESPONSE

1. Which of the following are recommendations from the American Academy of Pediatrics (AAP) for breast-feeding infants? Select all that apply.

    A. Newborns should be nursed when they begin crying.
    B. Healthy, term infants should remain in skin-to-skin contact with mothers beginning 12 hours after delivery.
    C. No supplements should be given to newborns unless a medical indication exists.
    D. Exclusive breastfeeding is ideal to support growth and development for approximately six months.
    E. Gradual introduction of iron-fortified foods should complement breastfeeding after six months.

2. Which of the following are true statements regarding the fat content of breast milk? Select all that apply.

    A. Fat content decreases during the day, with early morning milk having the highest fat content.
    B. Total fat content increases from colostrum to mature milk.
    C. The total fat content of human milk is approximately 15 percent.
    D. Fats found in breast milk support development of cell membranes in the body.
    E. Hindmilk contains more fat than foremilk.

3. Which of the following guidelines will ensure the most effective position for both mother and baby during breastfeeding? Select all that apply.

    A. The baby needs to be held close, supporting his back, shoulders, and neck.
    B. The breast should be brought to the baby; the baby should not be brought to the breast.
    C. There are a variety of positions used for breastfeeding; the most effective are based on mother's preference and condition.
    D. For best results, the mother should lie on her back with a pillow under her knees.
    E. The baby's head and body need to be in a straight line to make swallowing easier.

UNIT 7

Newborn Development and Nursing Care

CHAPTER 21

Transition to Extrauterine Life

KEY TERMS

Please define the following terms:

Asphyxia

Behavioral state

Congenital heart defects

Diaphragmatic hernia

Ductus arteriosus

Ductus venosus

Extrauterine life

Fetal circulation

Foramen ovale

Habituation

Hypoglycemia

Hypothermia

Hypovolemia

Meconium staining

Neutral thermal environment

Postnatal (or adult) circulation

Preterm

Primary apnea

Pulmonary vascular resistance (PVR)

Resuscitation

Secondary apnea

Sepsis

Thermoregulation

Transient tachypnea of the newborn (TTN)

ACTIVITIES

1. Describe the major factors necessary for the transition from intrauterine to extrauterine life.

2. Fluid within the lungs must be cleared during pulmonary transition. Explain how this is achieved.

3. Describe the significant effects of the first breath on cardiovascular function.

4. Identify the changes that occur in the cardiovascular system as a result of cord clamping and the loss of placental circulation.

5. Describe the major changes in thermoregulation that occur at the time of birth.

6. Explain the importance of brown fat in the newborn.

7. Explain the nursing process in maintenance of a neutral thermal environment for the infant.

8. Discuss the major change that occurs at the time of birth in the metabolic process.

9. Define the changes that occur in the neonate in regards to the gastrointestinal system.

10. Describe, in detail, the first few minutes after the birth of the infant and the changes that occur.

11. Describe the neurobehavioral transition of the newborn:

	First Period of Reactivity	Period of Decreased Activity	Second Period of Reactivity
Description			
Activity			
Time			
Implementation: newborn and family			

12. Compare primary and secondary apnea in the newborn.

13. Discuss the common complications of transition of the newborn:

    Asphyxia

    Meconium staining

    Transient tachypnea

    Hypoglycemia

    Hypovolemia

14. Describe the implications of a newborn's transition to extrauterine life if congenital heart defects are present.

15. Explain how viral or bacterial endotoxins affect a newborn's transition to extrauterine life.

16. Describe the complications of a diaphragmatic hernia and the rationale for immediate surgery.

17. Identify the complications of cardiac system transition.

18. In communicating with prospective parents of preterm neonates:

    a. Describe the information that should be discussed with the parents.

    b. Describe what terminology should be avoided with the parents.

19. List the indications for the use of resuscitation of an infant.

20. Describe medications and doses that may be used in resuscitation of the newborn.

SELF-ASSESSMENT QUIZ

1. Three fetal circulatory shunts, in utero, allow highly oxygenated blood to be diverted to the brain and heart. Identify them.

2. Describe the mechanism of the ductus venosus.

3. Describe the mechanism of the foramen ovale.

4. Describe the mechanism of the ductus arteriosus.

5. Describe the importance of surfactant in the respiratory system.

6. Identify the number of veins and arteries in the umbilical cord.

7. Once the placenta is removed, the neonate must change from a fetal circulatory pathway to which type of circulation?

8. What is the primary mechanism of heat energy production in the first days of life?

9. Identify the estimated heat loss of the infant in the delivery room.

10. Explain the effect of the infant's first breath on the gastrointestinal system.

11. Describe the "en face" position of the infant.

12. Describe the resuscitation measures of the newborn.

13. Identify the three major diseases that may impede the newborn's transition to extrauterine life.

14. Identify the number of skilled caregivers that should be available when a healthy newborn is anticipated and when a problem is anticipated.

15. State the indications of positive pressure ventilation on an infant at birth.

16. True or False

    T   F   Meconium staining rarely occurs in infants born after 34 weeks' gestation.

    T   F   Postnatal circulation of the newborn resembles adult circulation.

    T   F   The ductus arteriosus connects the umbilical vein to the inferior vena cava.

    T   F   The first breath the infant takes results in the following cardiovascular changes: the pressure in the right side of the heart falls and pulmonary venous return increases to the left atrium.

T F The majority of brown fat in the infant is located around the blood vessels and muscles in the neck, clavicles, axilla, and sternum.

T F Newborn glucose levels begin to stabilize by one to three hours.

T F The first point at which respiration is possible in the premature infant is 24 to 26 weeks' gestation.

CRITICAL THINKING

Ms. S. is happily showing off her newborn son to all her visitors. Baby Joey was born six hours ago. When you perform your assessment, you discover his axillary temperature is only 97.2°F.

1. What factors could place this infant at risk for hypothermia?

2. What additional assessments would you perform at this time?

3. After you stabilize Joey's temperature, develop a teaching plan for his parents.

MULTIPLE CHOICE

1. Which of the following is a true statement regarding the transition of the newborn's gastrointestinal system to extrauterine life?

   A. The infant's abdomen is typically full and rounded at birth, transitioning to flat.
   B. Bowel sounds become audible by stethoscope within the first 15 minutes after birth.
   C. The infant will pass meconium for the first time after approximately 12 to 24 hours.
   D. The gastrointestinal tract in the extrauterine environment is almost identical to the gastrointestinal system in the intrauterine environment.

2. Two neurobehavioral competencies that provide information regarding the infant's adjustment to extrauterine life are _____ and _____.

   A. reactivity, regulation
   B. alertness, organization
   C. infant state, habituation
   D. situation, determination

3. During an initial assessment after birth, the nurse notices the infant's heart rate is beginning to fall, his blood pressure is elevated, and he is not breathing. What is the nurse's assessment and treatment at this point?

   A. The infant is in primary apnea and should be stimulated to breathe by rubbing his back and providing free-flow oxygen.
   B. The infant is in primary apnea and should be given oxygen through positive pressure ventilation.
   C. The infant is in secondary apnea and should be stimulated to breathe by rubbing his back and providing free-flow oxygen.
   D. The infant is in secondary apnea and should be given oxygen through positive pressure ventilation.

4. Which of the following is a true statement regarding positive pressure ventilation?

    A. Positive pressure ventilation should be initiated any time the heart rate falls below 120 bpm.
    B. The best type of positive pressure ventilation for an infant with a diaphragmatic hernia is bag-mask ventilation.
    C. Positive pressure ventilation should be administered at a rate of 20 to 40 breaths per minute.
    D. Ineffective ventilation may be caused by an improper seal or the presence of the newborn's secretions.

5. Which of the following medications administered during neonatal resuscitation can be given through the endotracheal tube?

    A. naloxone hydrochloride
    B. epinephrine
    C. sodium bicarbonate
    D. Ringers' lactate

MULTIPLE RESPONSE

1. Which of the following are true statements regarding the newborn's cardiac system transition from intrauterine to extrauterine life? Select all that apply.

    A. The foramen ovale closes after diminished right-to-left shunting between the atria.
    B. Blood flow through the ductus arteriosus reverses and blood flows from right to left.
    C. Functional closure of the ductus arteriosus occurs within approximately 30 minutes after birth.
    D. The ductus venosus constricts after birth as blood stops flowing through the umbilical vein.
    E. Functional closure of the ductus venosus occurs within two to three days.

2. Which kinds of newborn activities can a parent expect to see during the first period of reactivity? Select all that apply.

    A. slow heart rate and deep respirations
    B. a state of alertness
    C. high muscular tone
    D. sucking, chewing, and rooting activities
    E. crying and fussiness

3. Which of the following is a potentially chronic complication associated with prematurity? Select all that apply.

    A. lung disease
    B. periventricular leukomalacia
    C. hydrocephalus
    D. sepsis
    E. patent ductus arteriosus

CHAPTER 22

Nursing Care of the Normal Newborn

KEY TERMS

Please define the following terms:

Acrocyanosis

Anal wink reflex

Anterior fontanel

Caput succedaneum

Cephalhematoma

Chorioamnionitis

Coarctation of the aorta

Cyanosis

Developmental dysplasia of the hip (DDH)

Erythema toxicum

Imperforate anus

Lanugo

Macrocephaly

Meconium

Microcephaly

Milia

Mongolian spots

Mottling

Patent ductus arteriosus (PDA)

Polydactyly

Posterior fontanel

Postterm

Preterm

Pustular melanosis

Syndactyly

Tachycardia

Tachypnea

Term

ACTIVITIES

1. Identify the alternative method of producing body heat in the newborn.

2. Describe the events the nurse monitors in the newborn's cardiovascular system.

3. The nurse identifies the characteristics of peripheral pulses. Describe them.

4. Describe the observations the nurse must make in evaluating the infant's respiratory effort.

5. Describe choanal atresia.

6. Explain the rationale for ophthalmic prophylaxis.

7. Define the rationale for prophylactic injections of vitamin K to the infant and the possible results if not given.

8. State the purpose of the numerous newborn assessments completed by the nurse in the first four to six hours of life.

9. Differentiate between jaundice that appears prior to and after 24 hours of age.

10. Nurses examining the skin of newborns should pay particular attention to which parts of the body?

11. Explain the importance of reactivity in relationship to the neuromuscular system.

12. Describe identification of the newborn and required security procedures.

13. State the rationale for plotting the infant's weight, length, and head circumference.

14. Describe normal vital signs and average weight, length, and head circumference of the newborn.

15. Calculate the following of a newborn:

    Infant length 21 inches=_____ cm

    Infant length 19 1/2 inches=_____ cm

    Infant weight eight pounds=_____ grams

    Infant weight six and a half pounds=_____ grams

16. Describe the assessment of the following 12 newborn characteristics:

    Posture

    Square window

    Arm recoil

    Popliteal angle

Scarf sign

Heel to ear

Skin

Lanugo

Plantar surface

Breasts

Eye and ear

Genitalia

17. Describe the assessment of the following systems in the newborn:
Integumentary

Head, ears, eyes, nose, throat (HEENT)

Respiratory

Cardiovascular

Abdomen

Genitalia and anus

Musculoskeletal

Neurologic

Body size classification

18. Describe all the elements of the integumentary system.

19. Discuss the variation in the integumentary system noted in newborns.

20. State the areas on the newborn a nurse may examine to determine meconium staining.

21. Differentiate birthmarks from marks that result from trauma to the infant during the birthing process.

22. Define the difference between a blue or blue-black birthmark and a Mongolian spot.

23. Describe the visual inspection the nurse utilizes for the head, ears, eyes, nose, and throat.

24. Differentiate the anterior fontanel from the posterior fontanel.

25. Differentiate caput succedaneum from cephalhematoma.

26. Discuss the importance of the absence of the red reflex to the newborn's eye.

27. List the characteristics noted in an infant with Down syndrome.

28. Describe the physical and mental effects on the newborn due to alcohol-related birth defects and fetal alcohol syndrome.

29. Describe common problems related to the respiratory system noted in the newborn.

30. Describe the cardiovascular system examination and assessment by the nurse.

31. Discuss the common variations of the cardiovascular system in the newborn.

32. Discuss the common problems of the cardiovascular system noted in the newborn.

33. Describe the examination of the newborn's abdomen. Include the umbilical cord and bowel sounds.

34. Discuss the common variations found in the newborn abdomen.

35. Describe the common problems seen in the newborn abdomen.

36. Explain the anal wink reflex.

37. Summarize the concerns of the nurse in finding blood in the following locations on the diaper of a newborn:

    Near the top

    Middle (female)

    Middle (male)

38. Discuss the common problems associated with male and female genitalia.

39. Describe imperforate anus.

40. Discuss the acronym VATER.

41. Summarize the risks and benefits of circumcision in the infant boy.

42. Describe the instructions a nurse would give to parents of a newborn male with a circumcision.

43. Describe visual inspection of the musculoskeletal system.

44. Discuss the common variations of the musculoskeletal system.

45. Discuss common problems in the musculoskeletal system.

46. Explain Ortolani's maneuver.

47. Define a simian crease.

48. Describe periodic shift assessment. Identify the assessments made, and list findings to be reported to the medical staff.

49. Discuss quick examination.

50. Describe interactional assessment.

51. Describe the psychological conditions that place an infant at risk.

52. Identify assistance that the nurse may arrange for the family and the newborn.

53. Identify environmental factors that could put the newborn at risk upon discharge.

54. Define the maternal illness that could be detrimental to the newborn and possibly lead to sepsis.

55. Discuss Erikson's first developmental stage of trust versus mistrust and the newborn.

56. Describe the importance of sleep and activity in the newborn.

57. Develop a plan for parents to follow in regards to cord and skin care upon discharge for the newborn.

58. Identify two criteria necessary for discharge of the newborn.

SELF-ASSESSMENT QUIZ

1. Explain the measures taken to assist the newborn in maintaining body temperature and to prevent chilling.

2. Axillary infant temperatures should be maintained where?

3. State a cause of transient tachypnea of the newborn.

4. A two-vessel umbilical cord (one vein, one artery) could be associated with what anomalies?

5. Describe hemolytic and physiologic jaundice.

6. A pink skin color on all infants indicates _____.

7. A decrease of 10 mmHg or more in the thigh in comparison to the arm, or a systolic blood pressure of more than 90 mmHg, is indicative of what anomaly?

8. Identify the weeks' gestation with the following term:

   Preterm

   Term

   Post-term

9. Compare erythema toxicum and Mongolian spots.

10. What changes in birthmarks are parents taught to observe and report?

11. Identify the common areas to inspect for birth injuries.

12. The presence of petechiae on infant skin not attributed to birth injury could represent what?

13. Describe the characteristics of a coloboma in a newborn.

14. State the first visual assessment of the respiratory system made by the nurse.

15. Describe the normal heart rate of a newborn. Also describe tachycardia.

16. Describe the signs of infection in a circumcision.

17. Explain achondroplasia and describe this condition.

18. Differentiate between polydactyly and syndactyly.

19. Identify the parameters to determine size classification using weight, length, and head circumference measurements.

CRITICAL THINKING

Jane delivered a nine-pound baby girl, Chyna, following a 16-hour labor. The second stage of labor lasted almost three hours and forceps were required. Twenty-four hours later you observe that baby Chyna's skin is jaundiced.

1. What further assessments would you perform at this time?

2. What are the common risk factors for pathological newborn jaundice?

3. Jane is very interested in caring for her daughter and expresses concern about her baby's umbilical cord. Jane asks how to bathe her baby before the cord falls off. Write a teaching plan to assist Jane with the cord care of her daughter.

MULTIPLE CHOICE

1. A nurse is performing an initial assessment on an infant and notices that large bubbles are appearing around the mouth and coming out of the nose. What is the nurse's first response?

   A. do nothing; this is a normal infant behavior
   B. suction the mouth and nose with a bulb syringe
   C. provide free-flow oxygen at 5 L/min
   D. notify the pediatrician

2. The assessment test that involves pressing the infant's wrist and palm toward the forearm is known as _____.

   A. popliteal angle   C. square window
   B. arm recoil   D. scarf sign

3. Which of the following is considered to be a normal finding when assessing the integumentary system of a newborn?

   A. port wine stain   C. hair over the forehead
   B. plethora   D. pustular melanosis

4. Which of the following is a risk associated with circumcision?

   A. skin dehiscence   C. increased risk of penile cancer
   B. urinary tract infection D. inguinal hernia

5. Which type of assessment involves taking the infant's vital signs, body weight, feeding and elimination details, and assessing respiratory and cardiac function?

   A. quick examination   C. periodic shift assessment
   B. body size classification D. interactional assessment

MULTIPLE RESPONSE

1. Which of the following are true statements related to a newborn's temperature control? Select all that apply.

   A. The skin occupies the largest surface area, causing heat loss by evaporation.
   B. Infants who are chilled are not able to produce body heat by shivering.
   C. A rectal temperature provides the most accurate result when measuring infant body temperature.
   D. Infants have a thick, subcutaneous layer of fat that provides a little warmth.
   E. To maintain body temperature, an infant should be placed in a radiant warmer or in skin-to-skin contact with the mother.

2. Which of the following are factors that may help to prevent infant abductions? Select all that apply.

   A. All nursing staff and personnel are identified specifically by the clothes they wear.
   B. When the mother is ill, the infant may also be left with a grandmother.
   C. The mother's written permission is required for family to hold or feed the infant while under the nurse's care.
   D. The identity of the mother of the newborn is verified by the institution's device for identification.
   E. Transportation of infants from one nursing unit to another should by done only by authorized nursing staff.

3. Which of the following are considered to be common findings encountered when assessing the genitalia of a newborn? Select all that apply.

   A. bruising of the scrotum
   B. vernix caseosa
   C. smegma under the foreskin
   D. hood-shaped clitoris
   E. hymenal tag

CHAPTER 23

Care of Newborns at Risk Related to Birth Weight and Premature Delivery

KEY TERMS

Please define the following terms:

Apnea

Asymmetric IUGR

Auditory brain evoked response (ABER)

Bilirubin

Bronchopulmonary dysplasia (BPD)

Containment

Developmental care

Dysmotility

Extremely low birth weight (ELBW)

Gastroesophageal reflux (GER)

Gavage feeding

Glycosuria

Hyaline membrane disease (HMD)

Hyperglycemia

Hyperkalemia

Hypernatremia

Hypoglycemia

Hyponatremia

Insensible water loss (IWL)

Intrauterine growth restriction (IUGR)

Intraventricular hemorrhage (IVH)

Jaundice

Large for gestational age (LGA)

Low birth weight (LBW)

Macro-environment

Micro-environment

Necrotizing enterocolitis (NEC)

Neutropenia

Oliguria

Opsonization

Osteopenia

Patent ductus arteriosus (PDA)

Perinatal asphyxia

Persistent pulmonary hypertension in the newborn (PPHN)

Plethora

Pneumatosis intestinalis

Postconceptional age

Posthemorrhagic hydrocephalus

Prematurity

Preterm birth

Respiratory distress syndrome (RDS)

Retinopathy of prematurity (ROP)

Short bowel syndrome

Small for gestational age (SGA)

Symmetric intrauterine growth retardation (IUGR)

Total parenteral nutrition (TPN)

Ventricular peritoneal shunt (VPS)

Very low birth weight (VLBW)

ACTIVITIES

1. Infants born SGA are at high risk for multiple problems. List them.

2. Explain the use of ultrasonography in establishing the predelivery diagnosis of IUGR.

3. Describe in detail the care given to an infant who upon birth is determined to be SGA.

4. Discuss the outcome and follow-up including the mortality risk for an SGA infant.

5. Describe associated factors of infants that may lead to being LGA.

6. Identify possible complications for infants who are LGA.

7. List the risk factors associated with preterm labor and delivery.

8. List the factors that occur during pregnancy that put a woman at risk for preterm labor and delivery.

9. Describe gestational age assessment and its importance in anticipating problems.

10. Identify the risk factors for the mother associated with preterm labor and delivery.

11. Identify the risk factors for the infant associated with preterm labor and delivery.

12. Describe the physical characteristics of a premature infant. Compare the characteristics with gestational age.

13. Define the cause, treatment, symptoms, and diagnosis of a premature infant with PDA.

14. Describe the effects of hypotension on the premature infant.

15. Define IVH and its effects on the premature infant.

16. After IVH, posthemorrhagic hydrocephalus may develop. State the signs, symptoms, and treatment.

17. Define hearing impairment in the premature infant and list the associated risk factors.

18. Differentiate between acute and physiologic anemia.

19. Describe the etiology, effects, and treatment of hyperbilirubinemia. Give the reason the premature infant is at increased risk.

20. Define the following in association with NEC:
    Characteristic

    Prevention

    Etiology

    Predisposing factors

    Early symptoms

    Second stage of symptoms

    Late onset symptoms

    Treatment

    Laboratory evaluation

Surgical interventions

Complications

Late complications

21. Describe the risks associated with the immune system in the premature infant.

22. Compare maternal and neonatal risk factors in infection.

23. Define the nurse's role in caring for premature infants for the prevention of infection.

24. The skin of the premature infant is fragile. Describe the following and their effects on the neonate:
    Epidermal stripping

    Absorption of chemical agents

    Intravenous fluid infiltrates

25. Discuss the risk to the premature infant's ophthalmologic system, including the following:
    ROP

    Retinal detachment

    Other eye problems such as myopia, amblyopia, glaucoma, and strabismus

26. Discuss oliguria and glycosuria in the premature infant.

27. Summarize the respiratory system of the fetus.

28. Describe RDS in the premature infant.

29. Discuss BPD, the focus of nursing care, and the importance of the family for the premature infant.

30. Discuss apnea in the premature infant.

31. Describe special considerations in the care of the high-risk infant. Include the parental challenge and nursing considerations.

32. Define the ethical considerations and goals involved in care of the premature infant.

33. Explain fluid loss of the preterm infant, including the following:
    Insensible water loss

    Overall goals of fluid management

    TPN

    VLBW

    ELBW

34. Discuss electrolyte management in the preterm infant, including hyponatremia, hypernatremia, and hyperkalemia.

35. Define hypoglycemia and hyperglycemia in regards to the premature infant.

36. Differentiate between formula feeding and breastfeeding for the premature infant.

37. Explain pain management in the neonate.

38. Discuss the importance of touch and massage to the preterm infant.

39. Describe the benefits of skin-to-skin holding for the preterm infant.

40. Co-bedding of twins has been found to be positive. Evaluate the effects.

41. Describe the importance of the neonatal transport team.

42. Describe the environment of a neonatal intensive care unit (NICU).

43. Compare the macro-environment and the micro-environment.

44. Describe the effects of nursery light on the vision system of an infant. Does this affect other aspects of the preterm infant's functioning?

45. List strategies for reducing the effects of light on the infant in the NICU environment.

46. List five ototoxic drugs that an infant may receive during hospitalization.

47. Compare the sound level in the NICU to sound levels in the environment.

48. Discuss the effects of NICU sound levels on a preterm infant's hearing.

49. Propose interventions to decrease the sound level in the NICU setting.

50. Explain why premature infants are vulnerable to the effects of environmental temperature.

51. How is heat lost in the high-risk infant?

52. Discuss interventions for reducing heat loss in an infant.

53. Propose a client education plan for parents learning how to position their new infant.

54. Discuss the postural disorders common to chronically ill, preterm neonates.

55. Discuss interventions for developmentally supportive positioning for infants.

56. Discuss strategies to organize nursing care to provide adequate rest for preterm infants.

57. Explain the concept of kangaroo care.

58. Discuss the positive outcomes nonnutritive sucking provides for preterm infants.

59. Propose interventions to provide nonnutritive sucking for infants.

SELF-ASSESSMENT QUIZ

1. List the causes of asymmetric IUGR.

2. List the factors that may affect fetal growth.

3. List the maternal factors that may affect fetal growth.

4. Describe the symptoms associated with hypotension as seen in the newborn infant.

5. Describe the symptoms associated with a premature infant born with **PDA**.

6. Identify the common problems associated with the neurological system as seen in the premature infant.

7. At _____ weeks' gestation, peristalsis begins to occur.

8. Differentiate between protein and carbohydrate absorption in the premature infant.

9. State the reasons the premature infant is at risk for GER.

10. Describe the four mechanisms the newborn uses to produce heat.

11. Name the four modes of heat transfer by which an infant can lose heat.

12. True or False

    T   F   LBW infants are defined as infants weighing more than 2,500 grams.

    T   F   IUGR is a term used for infants who, on standardized graphs, are less than 20% at birth in weight, length, and head circumference.

    T   F   Asymmetric IUGR is less likely to be caused by extrinsic factors than is symmetric IUGR.

    T   F   Outcomes are better in infants who have asymmetric IUGR compared with those who have symmetric IUGR.

    T   F   Placental insufficiency is the leading cause of SGA infants.

    T   F   A premature infant is an infant born before 37 weeks' gestation.

    T   F   Motility of the gastrointestinal tract changes during gestation and birth.

    T   F   The more premature the infant, the greater the delay in passage of stool.

    T   F   The most common risk factor for infection in the preterm infant is exposure to infection in utero.

    T   F   The placenta acts as the organ of respiration for the fetus in utero.

    T   F   The main substance necessary for energy, brain metabolism, and central nervous system integrity is potassium.

    T   F   One of the earliest interventions known to improve survival in premature infants was maintaining a warm environmental temperature.

13. List two categories of drugs commonly used in the NICU setting that may be ototoxic.

CRITICAL THINKING

Baby girl Sara's gestational age is 36 weeks, and her weight of 1,500 g places her below the tenth percentile for weight. This infant's weight and gestation classify her as both SGA and premature. When Sara's mother was 34 weeks' gestation she was diagnosed with pregnancy-induced hypertension. Although the mother received good prenatal care, she continued to smoke one pack of cigarettes each day. She denied any alcohol use.

  1. List which factors affect growth potential of the fetus.

  2. Which factors in this mother's history put her at increased risk for giving birth to an SGA baby?

3. There are unique problems associated with SGA babies. List the possible complications for this baby.

4. When you assess the baby you notice abdominal distension and blood in her stool. What serious complication would you suspect?

5. Which intervention would have the highest priority at this time and why?

MULTIPLE CHOICE

1. An infant with an intraventricular hemorrhage that affects the subependymal germinal matrix would be classified as Grade _____.

    A. I   C. III
    B. II   D. IV

2. Which of the following is a potential negative outcome associated with betadine absorption through the skin of a neonate?

    A. central nervous system damage   C. transient hypothyroidism
    B. sloughing of the skin   D. increased blood alcohol levels

3. Which of the following is a method of preventing bronchopulmonary dysplasia?

    A. vitamin D supplementation   C. closure of the ductus venosus
    B. administration of surfactant   D. free-flow oxygenation

4. Which of the following is a true statement regarding apnea of prematurity?

    A. Apnea may be classified as central or neurological.
    B. It is extremely important to promote neck flexion while positioning.
    C. Intervention includes gentle, tactile stimulation, such as stroking the foot.
    D. Medications for treatment are used to depress the chemoreceptors in the central nervous system.

5. Which of the following is a true statement regarding fluid management in the neonate?

    A. The preterm infant's total body water is 90-95%.
    B. Fluid losses are directly proportional to weight and gestational age.
    C. Decreased creatinine indicates renal problems due to prematurity.
    D. Weight loss is necessary and expected in the first few days of life.

MULTIPLE RESPONSE

1. Which of the following are signs of an intraventricular hemorrhage? Select all that apply.

   A. hyperglycemia
   B. apnea
   C. tachycardia
   D. seizures
   E. hyperbilirubinemia

2. Which of the following measures are taken for management of necrotizing enterocolitis (NEC)? Select all that apply.

   A. administering vitamins to boost the infant's immune system
   B. gastric decompression with an orogastric tube
   C. abdominal ultrasound every 24 hours
   D. measurement of intake and output
   E. administering antibiotics as ordered

3. Which of the following situations may make an infant more likely to develop glycosuria? Select all that apply.

   A. hyperbilirubinemia
   B. high blood pressure
   C. infection
   D. steroid administration
   E. intraventricular hemorrhage

CHAPTER 24

Care of Newborns at Risk Related to Congenital and Acquired Conditions

KEY TERMS

Please define the following terms:

ABO incompatibility

Acquired disorder

Anencephaly

Brachial palsy

Choanal atresia

Cleft lip

Clubfoot (talipes equinovarus)

Congenital disorder

Congenital heart defects (CHD)

Developmental dysplasia of the hip (DDH)

Diaphragmatic hernias

Encephalocele

Epispadias

Erythroblastosis fetalis

Esophageal atresia (EA)

Exstrophy of the bladder

Extracorporeal membrane oxygenation (ECMO) therapy

Facial palsy

Gastroschisis

Genetic disorder

Hydrocephaly

Hydrops fetalis

Hyperbilirubinemia

Hypocalcemia

Hypoglycemia

Hypomagnesemia

Hypospadias

Imperforate anus

Infant of a diabetic mother (IDM)

Intracranial hemorrhage (ICH)

Jaundice

Kernicterus

Macrosomia

Maternal sensitization

Meningocele

Microcephaly

Myelomeningocele

Omphalocele

Palate

Pathologic jaundice

Phototherapy

Physiologic jaundice

Polycythemia

Rh incompatibility

Sepsis

Spina bifida

Subarachnoid hemorrhage

Subdural hemorrhage

TORCH

Tracheoesophageal fistula (TEF)

ACTIVITIES

1. Differentiate among congenital disorders, genetic disorders, and acquired disorders.

2. Discuss the American Academy of Pediatrics recommendations for folic acid requirements and supplements.

3. What does the mnemonic TORCH stand for?

4. Compare the following central nervous system (CNS) anomalies:

Anomaly	Description	Signs and Symptoms	Prognosis	Treatment
Anencephaly				
Microcephaly				
Hydrocephaly				
Spina Bifida				

5. List the clinical manifestations of increased intracranial pressure.

6. Discuss the nursing care for a neonate with a CNS anomaly.

7. Describe choanal atresia.

8. Explain the physical assessment findings that may indicate the presence of a diaphragmatic hernia. What nursing interventions are indicated?

9. Discuss the assessment and interventions for an infant with CHD.

10. Design a client education plan for parents of an infant with CHD.

11. Discuss nursing care for an infant with a cleft lip or cleft palate.

12. Describe the postoperative care for an infant with a cleft lip or cleft palate.

13. Define the acronyms VATER and VACTERL.

14. Describe the nursing care for an infant with esophageal atresia and tracheoesophageal fistula.

15. Differentiate hypospadias and epispadias.

16. Explain how gender is assigned for an infant with ambiguous genitalia.

17. Discuss the following musculoskeletal anomalies:

Anomaly	Description	Signs and Symptoms	Diagnosis	Interventions
Developmental dysplasia of the hip				
Talipes equinovarus (clubfoot)				

18. Describe Ortolani's and Barlow's assessment tests.

19. What conditions are considered acquired disorders in the newborn?

20. What are the causes and results of palsy and paralysis?

21. Differentiate types of intracranial hemorrhage (ICH):

	Description	Signs and Symptoms	Diagnosis	Interventions
Subdural hemorrhage				
Subarachnoid hemorrhage				

22. Review the clinical problems for an IDM:

Problem	Definition	Findings	Interventions
Macrosomia			
Respiratory distress syndrome			
Hypoglycemia			
Hypocalcemia			
Hypomagnesemia			
Hyperbilirubinemia			
Polycythemia			

23. Compare and contrast physiologic jaundice and pathologic jaundice, including the treatment and nursing interventions for each.

24. Discuss RhoGam, including the indications, administration, and pharmacologic aspects.

25. Discuss safety concerns for an infant being treated for hyperbilirubinemia.

26. Differentiate between early-onset and late-onset sepsis of the newborn, including the diagnostic tests to confirm a diagnosis.

27. Describe the multidisciplinary approach for a newborn with a congenital disorder.

28. Propose a nursing care plan for a family and newborn with a congenital disorder.

SELF-ASSESSMENT QUIZ

1. When do the most common anomalies of the CNS occur during gestation?

2. What substance promotes neural tube closure?

3. List five manifestations of increased intracranial pressure in a newborn.

4. How long are infants obligate nose breathers?

5. When should gender be assigned in an infant with ambiguous genitalia?

6. Describe a positive Ortolani test.

7. What are common sites for newborn fractures?

CRITICAL THINKING

Mrs. K. is a 36-year-old gravida three para three who had a normal vaginal birth after a 23-hour labor. Baby Javier was born at 37 weeks' gestation, weighing nine pounds, three ounces. Mrs. K.'s two previous babies were each over nine pounds at birth. Gestational diabetes, polyhydramnios, and mild hypertension complicated this pregnancy.

1. List the fetal risk factors in an IDM.

2. What physical characteristics would you expect Javier to have?

3. Why is the IDM at increased risk for respiratory distress syndrome?

4. What are the most common congenital anomalies of an IDM?

5. What are Mrs. K.'s risk factors for developing gestational diabetes?

MULTIPLE CHOICE

1. Which of the following is a true statement about physiologic jaundice?

   A. Physiologic jaundice is typically evident in the first 24 hours of life.
   B. Physiologic jaundice affects approximately 15 percent of term newborns.
   C. Physiologic jaundice may occur due to conditions such as hypothyroidism or enzyme deficiencies.
   D. Physiologic jaundice often resolves without any intervention within six to seven days after birth.

2. The most common organism that causes sepsis in the newborn is _____.

   A. *Staphylococcus aureus*
   B. group B *Streptococcus*
   C. *Haemophilus influenza*
   D. *Listeria monocytogenes*

3. Which of the following is considered to be nursing care for the infant born with microcephaly?

   A. supportive care that assists parents with coping skills
   B. monitoring the infant for signs of increased intracranial pressure
   C. assisting with placement of a ventricular shunt
   D. educating parents about skin care and infection

4. A condition in which the bowel herniates through an abdominal wall defect to the right of the umbilicus is known as _____.

   A. omphalocele
   B. bowel exstrophy
   C. imperforate anus
   D. gastroschisis

5. The most common type of intracranial hemorrhage that often occurs due to trauma in the full-term infants is _____.

   A. subdural hemorrhage
   B. subarachnoid hemorrhage
   C. hydrocephalus
   D. kernicterus

MULTIPLE RESPONSE

1. Which of the following are considered clinical manifestations of increased intracranial pressure? Select all that apply.

   A. high-pitched, shrill cry
   B. lethargy
   C. "setting sun" sign
   D. sunken fontanels
   E. hyper-alert state

2. Which of the following are nursing care interventions for the infant born with spina bifida? Select all that apply.

   A. changing the infant's position every three hours to prevent pressure on a specific area
   B. assessing the infant for signs of increased intracranial pressure
   C. covering the sac with a moist, occlusive dressing
   D. manually emptying the bladder to stimulate urination
   E. performing passive range of motion exercises

3. Which of the following are true statements regarding an infant born with cleft lip and palate? Select all that apply.

   A. Cleft lip and palate is the most common craniofacial anomaly.
   B. Cleft lip occurs more commonly in females and is generally located on the right side.
   C. Infants with cleft palate are more prone to panic during feedings.
   D. Surgical repair of the cleft lip is performed at approximately three months of age.
   E. Cleft lip and palate is associated with other syndromes in approximately 50 percent of cases.

Answer Key

CHAPTER 1

Self-Assessment Quiz
1. F, T, T, F, T, T, F, T
2. Day hospitals
   Day surgery
   Transitional care units
3. Preferred provider organization (PPO)
   Health maintenance organization (HMO)
   Point-of-service plan (POS)
4. Allows for assessment, monitoring, and treatment of clients at a distance
5. Critical thinking skills include:
   Attainment of knowledge
   Ability to reason
   Analytic processing
   Clinical judgment
   Problem solving
   Critiquing
6. RhoGam is used when the Rh-negative mother is pregnant with an Rh-positive fetus.
7. Accuracy
   Thoroughness
   Compliance with standards
   Individualized nursing care based on client need
   Appropriate goals and interventions that are timely in completion
   Discharge planning
8. Pregnancy
   Delivery
9. Nurse midwife (women's health care), nurse practitioner, clinical nurse specialist and neonatal nurse practitioner

Critical Thinking
1. The Patient Protection and Affordable Care Act (PPAC) essentially requires that all Americans become insured. A portion of the plan includes for a provision to allow for insurance coverage for births that take place in birthing centers.
2. Women are more likely to live in poverty, or have low incomes both in single parent homes and older women as well. Lack of resources leads to a decrease in access to medical care and also affects the ability to promote health such as having the time to exercise.

Multiple Choice
1. B
2. D
3. A
4. D
5. C

Multiple Response
1. A, C, D
2. C, E
3. A, B, D, E

CHAPTER 2

Self-Assessment Quiz
1. F, F, T, F, T
2. The couple needs to work together to establish mutual roles related to discipline and take the time and energy to nurture their own relationship. All members of the blended family need to realize that establishing family rituals, traditions, and relationships will take time. All members need to establish dyadic relationships and learn to function as a family unit. Parents should help make noncustodial children feel they are a permanent part of the family. Parents should also take extra time for holiday planning, because there are additional relatives to consider. All members of the family must be flexible.
3. Women who feel they were surrounded by supportive people in labor report more positive feelings about their labor experience, use less pain medication, and are more likely to breastfeed than women who do not receive support during labor. In addition, these women experience less post-partum depression and report higher feelings of self-esteem.
4. Whenever possible, include the father in decision making. Provide ongoing communication. Coach the father with physical tasks to assist the mother, such as massaging her back. Encourage the father to cut the cord.

Critical Thinking
1. a. The stages of grieving are denial, anger, bargaining, resolution, and acceptance.
   b. Denial and anger; it's not uncommon for individuals to switch back and forth.
   c. Provide privacy. Allow time to hold and bond with baby. Provide mementos such as pictures, footprints, and bands. Respect any religious or cultural requirements.
2. Try to reschedule her appointments at a more convenient time. Research the possibility of a clinic nearer her home. Contact social services that have monies available for transportation. Provide emotional support and let the client know that she is a good parent. Let the client know you will work with her to help her solve this problem.
3. Personal opinion; responses will vary.

Multiple Choice
1. B
2. C
3. D
4. A
5. C

Multiple Response
1. C, D, E
2. A, B, E
3. B, C

CHAPTER 3

Self-Assessment Quiz
1. Traditional Chinese medicine—D
   Yoga—E
   Shamanic healing—A
   Ritual healing—B
   Ayurvedic medicine—C

2. T, T, T, T, T
3. Yes. It should be reported to the Food and Drug Administration.
4. Diagnosis and treatment of the musculoskeletal system and osteopathic manipulation therapy
5. St. John's wort

Critical Thinking
1. It is natural for clients to become discouraged with the medical model, especially when there is a lack of progress. As a general rule, the nurse should be supportive of complementary care as long as it is not harmful or does not interfere with traditional care. However, clients can easily be convinced to spend money on useless and perhaps harmful substances and need to be educated and cautioned about these risks.
2. In traditional Chinese medicine, moxibustion is used on people who have a cold or stagnant condition. In Western medicine, moxibustion has successfully been used to turn breech babies into a normal head-down position prior to childbirth. A landmark study published in the Journal of the American Medical Association in 1998 found that up to 75% of women suffering from breech presentations before childbirth had fetuses that rotated to the normal position after receiving moxibustion at an acupuncture point on the bladder meridian. Other studies have shown that moxibustion increases the movement of the fetus in pregnant women and may reduce the symptoms of menstrual cramps when used in conjunction with traditional acupuncture.
3. There are many reasons for a client not telling the provider about the use of complementary therapies. Some people harbor a distrust of traditional medicine. They fear their provider will discourage the use of anything that they cannot bill for. Some clients may feel embarrassed to report the use of complementary therapies to their providers. A client may also fail to comprehend the potential seriousness of a "natural remedy" and not understand the importance of disclosure.

Multiple Choice
1. C
2. A
3. B
4. C
5. D

Multiple Response
1. A, D, E
2. A, B, C
3. B, D, E

CHAPTER 4

Self-Assessment Quiz
1. Standards and Guidelines for Professional Nursing Practice in the Care of Women and Newborns published by the Association of Women's Health, Obstetric, and Neonatal Nurses
2. T, F, T, T, T

Critical Thinking
1. Validate the complexity of the clients' feelings and assist the clients with making an informed choice. The nurse must take care to not influence the clients based on her own values and ethics, but instead facilitate the best choice for the clients.
2. While the nurse has a duty to the institution, she has a greater legal and ethical responsibility to provide safe care to her clients. If the nurse believes she will be unable to provide safe, competent nursing care, she must not accept responsibility for the assignment. One solution would be to work with her supervisors in enlisting the help of other personnel.

Multiple Choice
1. B
2. D
3. A
4. B
5. C

Multiple Response
1. A, C
2. A, B, E
3. C, D, E

CHAPTER 5

Self-Assessment Quiz
1. 12 years of age
2. Heart disease
3. Anovulatory cycles account for 90 to 95 percent of dysfunctional uterine bleeding.
4. F, T, F, F
5. Alcohol and illicit drug use

Critical Thinking
1. a. Anorexia nervosa
   b. Ascertain Maria's self-image. Measure vital signs, height, and weight. Ask about any disruption of menstrual cycles.
   c. Anorexia is a potentially life-threatening condition. Maria must see a physician immediately, preferably someone with experience treating this disease.
2. a. Denial is a common reaction to abuse or violence. The nurse must ask directly if the client is suffering from abuse. Ask her about threats to herself or other members of her family, such as her children. Assure the client that anything she tells you will be held in confidence. If she is receptive, perform an abuse assessment.
   b. Provide her with the contact numbers of abuse hot lines and other community resources available.
   c. Client will not experience any physical or psychological violence or abuse. Client will develop a safety plan, which includes seeking out supportive family members and friends. Client will seek appropriate help from law enforcement and community resources.

Multiple Choice
1. B
2. C
3. D
4. A
5. C

Multiple Response
1. A, B, D
2. B, C, E
3. A, D

CHAPTER 6

Self-Assessment Quiz
1. White females
2. Coordinate women's health research funded by the NIH. Promote, stimulate, and support efforts to improve the health of women. Work in partnership with the NIH institutes and centers to

ensure that women's health research is part of the scientific framework at NIH. Strengthen and enhance research related to diseases, disorders, and conditions that affect women. Ensure that research conducted and supported by the NIH adequately addresses issues regarding women's health. Support research on women's health issues

3. Cardiovascular disease is the leading cause of death for both men and women.
4. Caucasian female
   Premature menopause
   Lack of exercise
   Excessive caffeine
   Regular alcohol use
   Excess dietary phosphate and sodium
   Menopause
   Calcium deficient diet
   Smoking
   Family history of osteoporosis
5. Over the age of 40
   Early menarche or late menopause
   Never having children
   Personal family history of breast cancer
   Atypical hyperplasia
6. Under the age of 25
   Having multiple sex partners without barrier protection
   Douching
   IUDs

Critical Thinking
1. a. Smoking, diet, and weight are all risk factors that can be modified
   b. Regular health check-ups, exercise, and walking
   c. Reduce or eliminate smoking, try low-fat recipes
   d. There is no one correct answer but "deficient knowledge R/T to cardiac risk factors" is an example of an appropriate nursing diagnosis
   e. Assist client in relating modifiable risk factors to herself. Discuss strategies for weight loss such as exercise and consuming a low-fat diet. Respect client's cultural and personal tastes with dietary intake. Assist client with smoking cessation programs.
2. Lifestyle changes such as smoking cessation, regular sleep habits, and stress reduction are some of the ways to reduce the symptoms of PMS.

Multiple Choice
1. C
2. B
3. B
4. D
5. A

Multiple Response
1. C, D, E
2. A, C, D, E
3. A, D, E

CHAPTER 7

Self-Assessment Quiz
1. Menarche
2. Onset is usually between the ages of 35 and 60. It is completed when the woman has completed one year without menses.

3. The disturbance of one or more of the phases of human sexual response. It may be biological, psychological, or social.
4. Permission
   Limited information
   Specific suggestions
   Intensive therapy
5. The inability to conceive after one year with appropriately timed coitus without the use of contraception.
6. The implantation of the uterine endometrium outside of the uterus. Endometriosis may cause infertility by obstructing implantation.
7. Relationships rather than objectivity
8. Reversible and permanent
9. Monophasic
   Biphasic
   Multiphasic
10. Decreased incidence of ovarian cancer; degree of protection increases with length of use (possibly 15 years). Reduced incidence of endometrial cancer; protection may last 15 years after discontinuance of medication.
11. Those who cannot take or do not tolerate estrogen, lactating women, and women with chronic medical conditions
12. Breakthrough bleeding
13. The client selection
14. The IUD works as an abortifacient.
    The IUD causes PID.
    The IUD causes ectopic pregnancies.
    Problems in past history of IUDs are common to all IUDs.
15. Delivers a child or has a substantial weight change
16. Do not use cornstarch or powders to store
    Vaginal lubricants should be water based. Petroleum products increase the risk of disintegration
    Must be positioned properly
17. Must fit properly
    Can remain in place 36 to 48 hours
    Must be left in place for six hours after intercourse because there may still be motile sperm
18. May be used for one to seven years depending on the product
    Requires minor surgery for insertion and removal
    Scar tissue may make it difficult to remove
19. Coitus interruptus—removal of the male penis from the vagina before ejaculation.
    Ovulation prediction (rhythm method)—the woman predicts her fertile period based on body temperature and/or cervical mucus changes.
20. Early in the cycle
21. Women—tubal ligation
    Men—vasectomy
22. F, T, T, F, T, F, F, T

Critical Thinking

1. During colonial times it was believed that the purpose of sexual relations was procreation. In the nineteenth century the focus of sexuality was on romance and intimacy. Contemporary attitudes ascribe to the belief that sexuality is linked to personal identity, individual desire, and personal fulfillment. The advent of modern contraception had a long-term and profound effect on modern sexuality. For the first time in history, a woman could choose when and if she were to become pregnant. Reliable, safe contraception allowed women to enjoy their sexuality without fear of unwanted pregnancy. A woman could be sexually active while pursuing a career or education. Marriage was less of a necessity and many couples chose to live together without the benefit of marriage.

Multiple Choice
1. C
2. B
3. D
4. C
5. A

Multiple Response
1. B, C, E
2. A, B, D
3. C, D, E

CHAPTER 8

Self-Assessment Quiz
1. Testosterone
2. Aortic fusiform or dissecting aneurysms
3. Third or fourth decade of life
4. Type III: sanfilipo
5. T, F, F, T
6. Trisomy 21—D
   Trisomy 13–15—A
   Trisomy 18—E
   XXY—B
   XYY—C
7. Drugs: antimalarial and aspirin
   Foods: fava beans

Critical Thinking
1. There is no right or wrong answer, just your personal feelings.
2. No right or wrong answer, just your personal views and feelings.
3. No right or wrong answer, just your personal feelings.
4. Pros: The knowledge would allow clients to make many important decisions regarding the disposition of their wealth and personal effects. They could choose not to have children due to the possibility of passing the disease on to the children as well as to consider the fact that they will most likely not be able to completely raise their children.
   Cons: Knowing what they have in store for them can remove all hope for a satisfactory life. Many clients experience extreme depression, and suicide is a major concern.

Multiple Choice
1. D
2. B
3. A
4. D
5. B

Multiple Response
1. B, E
2. A, B, D
3. C, D, E

CHAPTER 9

Self-Assessment Quiz
1. Quickening—C
   Fetal heartbeat by Doppler—B
   Ultrasound heartbeat—A
2. T, T, F, T, F, F
3. 12.5 kg/27.5 lbs.
4. A pregnant woman should not take any over-the-counter medications or complementary therapies without her primary care provider's permission. The client should increase dietary fiber, drink plenty of noncaffeinated fluids, exercise three to four times weekly, and maintain a normal bowel routine.
5. Exercise; avoid smoking, alcohol, and illicit drugs; get lomilomi massages; and follow a healthy diet.

Critical Thinking
1. There is a constant need for glucose for the developing fetus. Consequently, the pregnant woman produces more glucose, insulin, and triglycerides than a nonpregnant woman does. This places the woman in a diabetogenic state. These metabolic changes predispose pregnant women to gestational diabetes.
2. a. February eighth
   b. At the level of the umbilicus
   c. At approximately 20 weeks' gestation
   d. Provide reassurance to Mrs. Luna that softening and bleeding of the gums is a normal symptom of pregnancy. Estrogen causes increased proliferation of blood vessels and connective tissues in the gums.
   e. Teach Mrs. Luna the importance of always wearing seatbelts. The lap belt needs to be fastened under her belly and the shoulder belt should be fastened above her abdomen. She should never wear a seatbelt across her pregnant uterus.
   f. Although many women seek measures to either prevent stretch marks or cure them, there is no known medication or therapy for this normal condition. Her girlfriend most likely was not going to get stretch marks in any case.

Multiple Choice
1. B
2. D
3. A
4. B
5. C

Multiple Response
1. B, D, E
2. C, D, E
3. A, B, C

CHAPTER 10

Self-Assessment Quiz
1. Live virus or attenuated vaccines
2. F, T, F, T, F, F, T
3. B, A, A, A, B, B, A, B, A, B, A
4. gravida three, para three

Critical Thinking
1. a. Preterm labor

    Infections such as urinary tract infection or kidney infection (e.g., pyelonephritis)

    Normal back discomforts of pregnancy

    Back injury

  b. Description of pain and all related factors

    Presence or absence of vaginal discharge or bleeding

    Presence of dysuria, fever, or any other signs of infection

  c. Client most likely has an infection and will need to be seen by her provider immediately.
2. Responses will vary per individual.

Multiple Choice
1. D
2. B
3. C
4. A
5. D

Multiple Response
1. B, D, E
2. A, C, E
3. B, C, D

CHAPTER 11

Self-Assessment Quiz
1. Abruptio placenta
2. T, F, F, T, F, T, T, T
3. 72
4. A fasting blood sugar > 105 mg/dl or a two-hour postprandial glucose > 120 mg/dl
5. Experimentation with sexual relationships

   The need to love and be loved

   Peer pressure

   Promotion of self-esteem

   Partner pressure

   Need to feel grown up

   Loneliness

   Poor self-respect

   Alcohol

   Drug use
6. Adolescents younger than 16 years of age
7. Prenatally, during birth, and postnatally, during breastfeeding
8. Breastfeeding and nutrition

   Clothing and equipment needed

   Resources for well-child care

   Basic skills: bathing, diapering, and feeding

   How to take a temperature

   Recognition of urgent or emergent conditions

   Identification of emergency resources

   Auto and child safety

   Infant and child development

Critical Thinking
1. Vaginal bleeding in the early weeks of a probable pregnancy
   Mild hypotension and tachycardia indicate possible shock
   History of PID
2. History of PID from a chlamydia infection
3. A tubal pregnancy can rupture and lead to peritonitis and shock
4. Ultrasound and quantitative HCG testing

Multiple Choice
1. B
2. A
3. D
4. C
5. A

Multiple Response
1. A, B, C
2. A, B, E
3. C, D, E

CHAPTER 12

Self-Assessment Quiz
1. Mitosis refers to the process in which body cells duplicate themselves and then separate into two new daughter cells. This is how the human body grows and increases in size. It is the continuous process whereby the cell material duplicates and divides and is responsible for the growth of the fetus. Meiosis is the process by which the ovum and sperm divide and mature.
2. 23
3. F, T, F, F, F, F
4. The end of the eighth week
5. Refining structures and perfecting function
6. Embryonic stage—E
   3 weeks—A
   4 weeks—G
   5 weeks—B
   6 weeks—H
   7 weeks—C
   8 weeks—D
   9–12 weeks—M
   13–16 weeks—P
   17–19 weeks—L
   20–23 weeks—I
   24 weeks—N
   25–28 weeks—F
   29–32 weeks—J
   33–36 weeks—O
   38–40 weeks—K
7. X, A, B, C, D
8. Prenatal alcohol use
9. Toxoplasmosis
   Other infections including hepatitis
   Rubella
   Cytomegalovirus
   Herpes

10. Ductus arteriosus—D
    Ductus venous—C
    Foramen ovale—A
    Umbilical vein—B
11. Physicians, sonographers, laboratory technicians, and nurses
12. 40 weeks, 280 days after the first day of the last menstrual period

Critical Thinking
1. The nurse should ask opened-ended, nonjudgmental questions. Reassure the client that everything she tells you will be held in confidence. Discuss the possibility of sexual abuse.

Multiple Choice
1. B
2. B
3. C
4. A
5. C

Multiple Response
1. B, D
2. A, B, D
3. B, C, D

CHAPTER 13

Self-Assessment Quiz
1. Human chorionic gonadotropin, estrogen, estriol, and human placental lactogen
2. Late decelerations occur with less than half the uterine contractions.—C
   No late decelerations with three adequate uterine contractions in a ten-minute window, normal baseline fetal heart rate (FHR), and accelerations with fetal movement.—A
   Late decelerations occur with more than half the uterine contractions.—B
   Inadequate fetal heart rate (FHR) recording or less than three uterine contractions in ten minutes.—D
3. Biophysical profile
4. Suspected prematurity
   Suspected postmaturity
   Maternal diabetes mellitus
   Maternal hypertension: chronic and pregnancy-related disorders
   Suspected or documented intrauterine growth retardation
   Sickle cell disease
   History of previous stillbirth
   Isoimmunization
   Older gravida
   Chronic renal disease
   Decreasing fetal movement
   Severe maternal anemia
   Multiple gestation
   High-risk antepartal conditions

Critical Thinking
1. Increased maternal age at 37 years
   Family member with Down syndrome
2. Amniocentesis and quad screen
3. Explain that an amniocentesis is an outpatient procedure and obtain informed consent. Explain to the client her need for positioning and the process of the procedure. Stay with the client and provide support for anxiety.
4. Tell the client that some women experience a sensation of pressure or cramping.
5. Depending on test results and Mrs. B's statements, notify social services for assistance with decision making through the process. Outline all of the possibilities for continuation or termination of pregnancy for Mrs. B to decide. Contact a spiritual support person for counseling, if requested.

Multiple Choice
1. B
2. D
3. A
4. C
5. B

Multiple Response
1. A, B, E
2. B, C, E
3. A, B, D

CHAPTER 14

Self-Assessment Quiz
1.

Stage	Process	Time Element
1	Begins with the onset of labor and continues until full cervical dilation	Typically for prigravidas 12 hours; for multigravidas eight hours
2	Begins at the point of complete dilation of the cervix and is complete when the fetus is expelled	Primigravida 50 minutes Multigravida 20 minutes
3	Begins with the delivery of the fetus and ends with the delivery of the placenta and membranes	Usually eight to ten minutes following delivery of the neonate
4	Begins when the placenta and membranes are delivered	Complete four hours later

2. Labor induction, assisted delivery, augmentation, and cesarean section
3. Passageway or the birth canal
   Passenger, the fetus and placenta
   Powers, the uterine contractions
   Position of the mother
   Psychological response of the mother
4. False pelvis is the shallow upper section of the pelvis.
   True pelvis is the lower curved bony canal, including the inlet, cavity, and outlet through which the fetus must pass in the birth process.
5. Effacement is the shortening and thinning of the cervix. Cervical dilation is the widening of the cervical opening that occurs from myometrial contractions in labor.
6. Fontanels are the points of intersection of the skull bones. Molding is the overlapping of the fetal skull that helps the fetal head to adapt to the size and shape of the maternal pelvis.
7. Primary power is involuntary uterine contractions. Secondary power is the mother's intentional efforts to push out the fetus.

Critical Thinking
1. five to six hours
2. 0.5 to two mu/min.
3. Labor induction
   Labor augmentation
   Prevent or treat postpartum hemorrhage
4. Assess fetal heart tones
   Monitor uterine contraction patterns
   Assess vital signs, I&O
5. The oxytocin infusion is having the desired effect.
6. Turn off the oxytocin infusion.
   Open up the main IV to dilute oxytocin.
   Turn the mother on her side.
   Re-evaluate fetal heart tones and maternal blood pressure.

Multiple Choice
1. A
2. C
3. A
4. B
5. D

Multiple Response
1. B, D, E
2. A, B, E
3. A, D, E

CHAPTER 15

Self-Assessment Quiz
1. F, T, F, T, T, F
2. General anesthesia
   Cesarean delivery
   Blood transfusion and hysterectomy
3. Foods containing purines, such as organ meats, beer, and wine
4. The myometrium would be weaker and the client would have a higher-than-normal risk of uterine rupture.
5. Hypertension, diabetes, positive HIV, cardiac disease, phlebitis, renal disease, and seizure disorders
6. Information on the use of substances such as alcohol, tobacco, and illicit drugs can give clues to a client's lifestyle choices and health.
7. Frequency of a contraction is measured from the beginning of one contraction to the beginning of the next.
   Duration of a contraction is the time from the beginning of a contraction until the end of the same contraction.
8. Polyhydramnios is the presence of more than two liters of amniotic fluid.
   Oligohydramnios is less than 300 mLs of amniotic fluid in the uterus.
   At the end of pregnancy, the uterus contains 1,000 mL (one liter) of amniotic fluid.
9. Effacement is the taking up of the cervical canal from a thick, long structure to a paper-thin layer.
   Dilation is the widening of the external os of the uterine cervix from closed to a maximum of ten cm.
10. Dorsiflex the foot and ask the client if this causes calf pain. If so, this is a positive Homan's sign and should be further investigated.
11. Hypertension
    Proteinuria

12. Edema around the eyes
13. Albuminuria—possible complications, such as (PIH)
    Glucose—diabetes mellitus
    Ketones—inadequate nutrition
14. H&H—hematocrit and hemoglobin
    CBC—complete blood count
    HIV—human immunodeficiency virus
15. The fetal head is allowed to descend by means of involuntary uterine contractions (primary power).
16. Passive—the client does not have any urge to push.
    Active—pressure creates the urge to push, so the client should begin her expulsive efforts.
17. The fetal head passes under the pubic arch and the vertex is visible as it pushes the vaginal introitus open.
18. Episiotomy
19. The umbilical cord has become wound one or more times around the baby's neck.
20. An emergency in which the anterior shoulder cannot pass under the pubic arch after the fetal head is born.
21. Shallow regular breathing used 90% of the time.
    Deep irregular breathing used 10% of the time.
22. The hands and feet of the newborn are slightly blue; this condition may persist for seven to ten days.
23. One, five, and ten minutes
24. A full bladder
25. Uterus is not firm; may bleed more
26. At the level of the umbilicus
27. The bright red vaginal drainage the mother has after birth
28. Soft-tissue damage
    Retained products of conception (e.g., placental tissue or membranes)

Critical Thinking
1. There is a common perception that caring for a laboring client who is not using pharmacological relief is more difficult for the nurses.
2. Inform the coach of any progress or decisions.
   Involve the coach in decisions.
   Assist and support the coach with their role in the labor room.
3. Responses are individualized.

Multiple Choice
1. D
2. A
3. B
4. B
5. C

Multiple Response
1. B, D, E
2. A, B, D
3. A, C, D

CHAPTER 16

Self-Assessment Quiz
1. Oxytocin
2. T, F, T, T
3. Prematurity and low birth weight

Critical Thinking
1. Shoulder dystocia
2. Gestational diabetes
   Macrosomia
   Prolonged second stage
3. Remain with the physician or midwife and call for assistance
   Assist the physician or midwife with maneuvers
   Continually monitor the fetal heart rate
   Remain calm and facilitate the client's cooperation
   Notify the nursery
4. The client's legs are bent at the knees and hyperflexed against the abdomen to straighten the sacrum and alter the angle, allowing for the anterior shoulder to be dislodged.
   Suprapubic pressure consists of applying pressure either in an oblique or lateral approach or posteriorly and laterally, the anterior shoulder may be compressed and slip beneath the symphysis pubis.
5. Risk for hypoxia
6. Maternal injury and infection

Multiple Choice
1. B
2. C
3. A
4. B
5. D

Multiple Response
1. B, C, D
2. A, C, D
3. A, D, E

CHAPTER 17

Self-Assessment Quiz
1. First lumbar nerve (L1), second lumbar nerve (L2)
2. Local infiltration
3. Epidural
4. After the cuff of the endotracheal tube is inflated and placement has been verified

Critical Thinking
1. Mrs. M is experiencing pain due to cervical dilation and contraction of the uterus.
2. Position and movement, counter pressure, intradermal sterile water injection, birthing ball, hydrotherapy, heat and cold applications.
3. Intravenous analgesics, such as opiod narcotics; regional anesthesia, including epidural or spinal block.
4. If Mrs. M has not had regional anesthesia, local anesthesia would be provided to the site of the episiotomy to reduce pain. With regional anesthesia, the pain of an episiotomy may not be present during the procedure.
5. Monitor Mrs. M for signs of effective pain control following delivery and for nausea and vomiting, which are side effects of some types of analgesics. If regional anesthesia was used, assist Mrs. M with ambulating and instruct her to call before getting out of bed.

Multiple Choice
1. C
2. B
3. D
4. B
5. A

Multiple Response
1. B, D, E
2. A, B, E
3. A, B, C

CHAPTER 18

Self-Assessment Quiz
1. Puerperium—E
   Engorgement—I
   Residual urine—G
   Subinvolution—H
   Striae—J
   Lochia—K
   Involution—A
   Endometritis—C
   Atony—D
   Boggy uterus—B
   Episiotomy—F
2. Immediate—first 24 hours
   Early—second day to end of first week
   Ending—six weeks
3. Generally no difference
4. 12–15 pounds after delivery
   Five pounds during first week postpartum
   Ten pounds (approximate) in the next six weeks
5. Mother is Rh negative and gave birth to Rh-positive child; must receive RhoGam within 72 hours of delivery
6. Crying, sucking, smiling, clinging
7. 2, 3, 2, 3, 1, 1, 2, 2
8. T, T, F, T
9. Refer to infant by name
   Unwrap infant and initiate exploration of the infant's body
   Answer concerns the parents may have
   Encourage the mother to pick up and hold her infant
   Encourage the mother to hold her infant in the en face position
   Talk directly to the infant in a calm, soothing voice
   Utilize the infant's grasp reflex to hold onto the mother's finger
   Demonstrate comforting techniques, such as gentle patting and rocking

Critical Thinking
1. Marta is most likely in the taking-in period. Many new mothers spend a great deal of time in the immediate postpartum period retelling the events surrounding the birth.
2. The nurse should help the mother validate thorough active listening. Encourage her to verbalize her feelings.
3. Vital signs
   Breasts
   Uterus

Bladder
Bowel
Lochia
Episiotomy
Homan's sign
Emotional status

4. This would be an ideal time for Marta to receive a Rubella vaccine
5. Assist Marta to void, as a full bladder is the most common reason for a lateral deviation
6. Marta may require a pharmacological agent or she may be bleeding from a laceration in the birth canal
7. Uterine atony
   Retained placenta
   Cervical or perineal laceration
   Subinvolution
   Bleeding disorders

Multiple Choice
1. C
2. A
3. D
4. C
5. B

Multiple Response
1. A, C, E
2. B, C, D
3. B, E

CHAPTER 19

Self-Assessment Quiz
1. Oxytocin (Pitocin)
   Methylergonovine (Methergine)
   Carboprost tromethanmine
   Dinoprostone (misoprostol)
2. If the placenta is pulled out before it is ready to detach, uterine inversion, prolapse, or hemorrhage may occur. This is an emergency situation.
3. Uterine atony
4. Shock and numbness
   Searching and yearning
   Disorientation
   Reorganization
5. The mother who relinquishes her child experiences grief that may be prolonged; the nurse must be supportive of her decision.
6. Grief response
   Depression and grief
   Dysfunctional grieving
   Avoidance
   Prolonged and exaggerated grief
   Multiple loss
   Chronic grief
   Isolation

Critical Thinking

1. a. Liza may have a serious problem such as postpartum depression, psychosis, may simply be exhausted, or may feel responsible for her baby's prematurity.

   b. Because this may be a serious problem, the team should include nurses, physicians, social service, and psychiatric counselors.

   c. Explore the feelings and relevant symptoms the mother is experiencing, such as tearfulness, changes in appetite or sleep behaviors, the presence or absence of psychomotor agitation or retardation, fatigue or loss of energy, and any intrusive thoughts of death or suicide. Obtain pertinent information about Liza, such as a history of depression.

   d. Postpartum blues typically occur early in the postpartum period and are characterized by fatigue, tearfulness, and mild mood swings. Clients do not complain of feeling deep sadness nor experience any thoughts of death or suicide. Clients experiencing postpartum blues generally do well with explanations and support. PPD is a major depressive disorder, which is characterized by feelings of deep, unremitting sadness accompanied by many somatic and emotional complaints. Clients with PPD may have a history of depression, but many clients do not. PPD is a serious condition and may require psychotherapy, medications, and/or hospitalization. PPP is a rare serious psychiatric disorder. Symptoms often include extreme agitation, confusion, and inability to carry out activities of daily living, including infant care. Clients often experience auditory and visual hallucinations, and frequently experience ideations of suicide and death. The onset of PPP is a true emergency.

   e. Treatment often includes a hospitalization in a psychiatric facility and antipsychotic medications.

2. a. If fundus is boggy, provide fundal massage
   Assess vital signs, particularly blood pressure and pulse
   Be prepared to establish an intravenous access
   Be prepared to administer oxytocics

   b. Uterine atony
   Retained placenta
   Cervical or perineal laceration
   Subinvolution
   Bleeding disorders (e.g., disseminated intravascular coagulation)

Multiple Choice

1. B
2. A
3. B
4. D
5. C

Multiple Response

1. A, C, E
2. C, D, E
3. C, E

CHAPTER 20

Self-Assessment Quiz

1. 500
2. It is rich in antibodies and high in protein
3. T, T, F, F, T
4. Enzymes, proteins, fats, ions, water, and glucose
5. Transitional milk is produced following colostrum and immediately before mature milk. Foremilk is the thin, watery breast milk secreted at the beginning of a feeding. Hindmilk is the thick,

high-fat breast milk secreted at the end of a feeding that has the highest concentration of calories. It is thicker and richer in appearance.

Mature milk contains 10% solids for energy and growth.

6. Provides optimal nutrition, reduces risk for infectious diseases and other chronic conditions, provides unique positive interactions and bonding opportunities, and offers substantial health cost savings

7. Sucking movements, sucking sounds, hand-to-mouth movements, rapid eye movements, soft cooing sounds, fussiness

8. 1, 2, 2, 1, 1, 1, 2, 2

9. Six months of age

Critical Thinking

1. Any medical conditions that could affect success of breastfeeding
Diet and level of anxiety
Knowledge or experience related to breastfeeding

2. New research demonstrates that breast-feeding mothers return to prepregnant weight more quickly than bottle-feeding mothers.
Mother can be taught to express her breast milk into a bottle so that someone else can occasionally feed her infant.

3. Lactational amenorrhea, which promotes a longer period of decreased fertility
Less blood loss from amenorrhea
Improved remineralization
Reduction in hip fractures in postmenopausal period
Reduced rates of ovarian and premenopausal breast cancer
Promotes involution
Psychological benefits

4. Infant's gestational age
Any illness or congenital anomalies
Sucking reflex
Rooting reflex

5. Increases immunity and destroys pathogens
Breast milk supplies all of the nutrients to meet the ever-changing needs of the growing infant
Possible protective effect against sudden infant death syndrome, insulin dependent diabetes, lymphoma, and many other chronic illnesses
Breastfeeding has been shown to enhance intelligence and visual acuity

6. Transfer of maternal illness such as HIV or hepatitis infection
Abnormal anatomy of the breast, nipple inversion, or breast surgery may interfere with successful breastfeeding
Psychological barriers (e.g., modesty, fear, or lack of confidence)
Social barriers (e.g., lack of family support or an early return to work)

7. Short-term goals:
The client will express confidence in the ability to establish breastfeeding in first days postpartum
The infant will successfully latch-on the breast for each feeding
The client will demonstrate proper infant positioning
The client will discuss the amount and frequency of breastfeeding recommended
The client will remain free of severe breast pain during the early breastfeeding period
The client will express confidence in the ability to breastfeed at home
Long-term goals:
The client will successfully breastfeed the infant for at least six months
The infant will have a healthy and appropriate weight gain in the first six months of life

Multiple Choice
1. C
2. B
3. D
4. B
5. B

Multiple Response
1. C, D, E
2. B, D, E
3. A, C, E

CHAPTER 21

Self-Assessment Quiz
1. Ductus venosus
   Foramen ovale
   Ductus arteriosus
2. Connects the umbilical vein to the inferior vena cava; allows blood to bypass the liver.
3. Allows the blood entering the right atrium of the heart to go directly through the left atrium and out the ascending aorta to immediately supply the brain, heart, and upper extremities.
4. Shunts the blood from the pulmonary artery to the descending aorta, bypassing the lungs to perfuse the lower body, and return to the placenta for oxygenation.
5. Lowers the surface tension at an air-liquid interface.
   On expiration, the ability to retain air depends on surfactant.
   As surfactant lowers surface tension in the alveolus at end-expiration, it stabilizes the alveoli and prevents collapse.
6. Two arteries
   One vein
7. Postnatal (or adult) circulation
8. Brown fat metabolism
9. 0.4°F to 1.8°F per minute, depending on the infant's maturity and environmental conditions
10. When air is inspired, the intestinal tract begins to fill with air, the abdomen becomes more round and soft, and bowel sounds become audible. This usually occurs within the first 15 minutes of life.
11. The infant is placed in the parent's arms face-to-face to promote eye contact between parent and infant.
12. Emergency life support measures
    Airway management
    Positive pressure ventilation
    Chest compressions
    Medications
    Thermal support
13. Congenital heart defects
    Sepsis
    Diaphragmatic hernia
14. One caregiver should be present for a healthy newborn; two caregivers when a problem is anticipated.
15. Any time the heart rate is less than 100 bpm
    If the infant remains cyanotic despite 100% free-flow oxygen
16. F, T, F, T, T, F, T

Critical Thinking

1. The baby may be unwrapped in a cool room
   The baby is only six hours old
2. Complete set of vital signs
   Gestational status
   Room temperature
   How baby is dressed
3. Teach mom how to take Joey's axillary temperature
   Have parents demonstrate
   Avoid heat loss with appropriate clothing including a hat
   Swaddle infant in warm blankets
   Avoid placing Joey on a cold surface or near cool drafts
   Dry immediately after a warm bath

Multiple Choice

1. B
2. C
3. A
4. D
5. B

Multiple Response

1. A, D, E
2. B, C, D
3. A, B, C

CHAPTER 22

Self-Assessment Quiz

1. Place immediately in a temperature-controlled isolette or radiant warmer
   Swaddle in blankets and give stocking cap
2. 36.1°C to 37.5°C
   97°F to 99.5°F
3. Fluid remaining in the lungs
4. Renal and cardiac anomalies
5. Hemolytic jaundice is seen in the newborn infant less than 24 hours old and most likely results from serous blood incompatibilities between mother and infant.
   Physiologic jaundice is the gradual yellowing of the skin that may possibly have three nonhemolytic causes:
   Failure to adequately process bilirubin through inadequate intake or elimination
   Traumatic birth injuries
   Minor blood incompatibilities
6. Successful cardiac perfusion to the extremities
7. Coarctation of the aorta
8. Preterm—less than 37 weeks' gestation
   Term—between 37 and 42 weeks' gestation
   Post-term—beyond 42 weeks' gestation
9. Erythema toxicum is the most common skin eruption seen in newborns. It is a rash that occurs on the face and chest first and spreads to the rest of the body; the cause is unknown.
   There is no known treatment.
   Mongolian spots are normal variations in skin color that include dark blue, gray, or purple diffuse color seen on the buttocks of infants. They may also appear on the shoulders, forearms, and ankles. They fade and disappear as the child grows older.
10. Changes in color, shape, size, or elevation
11. Scalp, face, shoulders, arms, legs, and feet

12. An underlying infection, a hemorrhagic process, or a congenital condition (congenital rubella)
13. Examination of the iris of the eye shows what looks like a keyhole in the distant circle of the iris and pupil that will affect vision.
14. Symmetry of chest movements
15. Normal heart rate should fall between 120 and 150 bpm; heart rate above 160 bpm is tachycardia.
16. Failure to void adequately, bleeding from the operative site
17. Infants born with achondroplasia are referred to as dwarfs and have respiratory and neurologic problems in addition to skeletal defects. Characteristics include small thoracic cage, lack of the ability for elbow extension, and shortening of the humerus and femur.
18. Polydactyly—infant may have extra digits and toes.
    Syndactyly—digits and toes that appear to be linked together by webbing of the skin.
19. Small for gestational age (SGA) scores are under the 10th percentile.
    Appropriate for gestational age (AGA) scores are between the 10th and 90th percentile.
    Large for gestational age (LGA) scores are above the 90th percentile.

Critical Thinking
1. Blood type and presence of birth injuries
2. Trauma and hemolytic disease
3. Observe for oozing and bleeding at cord
   Notify provider if any bleeding or oozing is observed
   Observe for redness or pus and report if observed
   Fold diaper down for seven to ten days or until cord falls off
   Stump should dry for another five days
   Give baby sponge bath until cord falls off
   Demonstrate sponge bath and have mother return demonstration

Multiple Choice
1. B
2. C
3. D
4. A
5. C

Multiple Response
1. A, B, E
2. C, D, E
3. B, C, E

CHAPTER 23

Self-Assessment Quiz
1. Placental insufficiency
   Maternal malnutrition
   Extrinsic factors such as hypertension and low calorie intake
2. Normal variations such as race and gender
   Multiple gestation
   Chromosomal anomalies, such as trisomy 13 (Patau syndrome), trisomy 18 (Edwards' syndrome), and trisomy 21 (Down syndrome)
   Congenital malformations, such as anencephaly, gastrointestinal atresia, renal agenesis, cardiovascular defects, and congenital infection
   Rubella
   Cytomegalovirus
   Inborn errors of metabolism, such as transient neonatal diabetes, galactosemia, and phenylketonuria

3. Maternal hypoxia, such as sickle cell disease, respiratory disease, cardiovascular disease, and living in a high-altitude environment
   Short stature
   Young maternal age
   Low socioeconomic status
   Primiparity
   Grand multiparity
   Low pregnancy weight
   Maternal exposure to teratogenic agents, such as alcohol, cigarette smoking, and anticonvulsant medications
4. Tachycardia, pallor, poor capillary refill, poor peripheral pulses, and poor urine output
5. A murmur heard at the third intercostal space left of the sternal border, a hyperactive pericardium, bounding peripheral pulses, and a widening pulse pressure
6. Intraventricular hemorrhage
   Posthemorrhagic hydrocephalus
   Periventricular leukomalacia
   Hearing impairment
7. 28 to 30
8. Protein is handled well; carbohydrate absorption is limited because of lactose deficiency.
9. Immature muscle tone, poor sphincter control, delayed ion gastric emptying, and increased intra-abdominal pressure
10. Metabolic process
    Voluntary muscle activity
    Peripheral vasoconstriction
    Nonshivering thermogenesis
11. Evaporation
    Conduction
    Convection
    Radiation
12. F, F, F, T, T, T, T, T, T, T, F, T
13. Aminoglycosides and loop diuretics

Critical Thinking

1. Multiple gestation
   Gender and race
   Chromosomal abnormalities
   Maternal hypoxemia
   Sickle cell, any maternal illness
   Maternal smoking and alcohol consumption
   Placental insufficiencies
2. Pregnancy induced hypertension (PIH) can decrease placental perfusion
   Smoking decreases placental perfusion
3. Hypoxia
   Persistent pulmonary hypertension
   Meconium
   Hypothermia
   Hypoglycemia
   Hypocalcemia
   Hyperbilirubinemia
   Poylcythemia

4. Necrotizing enterocolitis
5. Immediately stop oral feeds to prevent peritonitis secondary to possible abdominal perforation. Begin an IV infusion to prevent dehydration.

Multiple Choice
1. A
2. C
3. B
4. C
5. D

Multiple Response
1. A, B, D
2. B, D, E
3. C, D, E

CHAPTER 24

Self-Assessment Quiz
1. Three to four weeks of gestation
2. Folic acid
3. Widening suture lines, bulging anterior fontanel, lethargy, irritability, high-pitched shrill cry, poor feeding, poor sucking, decreased level of consciousness, setting sun eyes, and opisthotonos
4. First three months of life
5. As soon as possible, preferably no later than two years of age
6. When a neonate's hip is flexed in a 90° angle, the leg is gently abducted, and an audible click is heard
7. Clavicle, humerus, femur, and skull

Critical Thinking
1. Macrosomia
   Respiratory distress
   Hypoglycemia
   Hypocalcemia
   Hypomagnesemia
   Hyperbilirubinema
   Congenital anomalies
2. Round chubby face, chubby body
   May be plethoric
   Much of the fat is distributed around head, chest, and shoulders
3. Hyperinsulinemia adversely affects surfactant production.
4. Cardiac and skeletal abnormalities
   Neural tube defects
   Delayed ossification
   Ventricular septal defect (VSD), coartation of the aorta
   Lazy colon syndrome
   Meningomyelocele and anencephaly
5. Infant weight over nine pounds: Large for gestational age
   Two previous babies born over nine pounds
   Polyhydramnios
   Mild hypertension

Multiple Choice
1. D
2. B
3. A
4. D
5. B

Multiple Response
1. A, B, C
2. B, D, E
3. A, C, D